T0275838

CAMBRIDGE LIBRARY COLLECTION

Books of enduring scholarly value

History of Medicine

It is sobering to realise that as recently as the year in which On the Origin of Species was published, learned opinion was that diseases such as typhus and cholera were spread by a 'miasma', and suggestions that doctors should wash their hands before examining patients were greeted with mockery by the profession. The Cambridge Library Collection reissues milestone publications in the history of Western medicine as well as studies of other medical traditions. Its coverage ranges from Galen on anatomical procedures to Florence Nightingale's common-sense advice to nurses, and includes early research into genetics and mental health, colonial reports on tropical diseases, documents on public health and military medicine, and publications on spa culture and medicinal plants.

Women as Army Surgeons

After training to be a doctor at the London School of Medicine for Women, Flora Murray (1869–1923) became an active member of the Women's Social and Political Union. At the outbreak of the First World War, she and her fellow suffragists laid down their banners and sought to aid the Allied war effort. Working within the newly formed Women's Hospital Corps, Murray and her colleague Louisa Garrett Anderson (1873–1943) overcame initial prejudice and established two military hospitals in France in the period 1914–15. Their success prompted an invitation from the War Office to open the Endell Street Military Hospital in London, staffed entirely by women. First published in 1920, Murray's account, illustrated with numerous photographs, records important steps in furthering the acceptance of women in the medical profession. For female doctors, surgeons and nurses, the war provided not only the 'occasion for service' but also 'great professional opportunities'.

Cambridge University Press has long been a pioneer in the reissuing of out-of-print titles from its own backlist, producing digital reprints of books that are still sought after by scholars and students but could not be reprinted economically using traditional technology. The Cambridge Library Collection extends this activity to a wider range of books which are still of importance to researchers and professionals, either for the source material they contain, or as landmarks in the history of their academic discipline.

Drawing from the world-renowned collections in the Cambridge University Library and other partner libraries, and guided by the advice of experts in each subject area, Cambridge University Press is using state-of-the-art scanning machines in its own Printing House to capture the content of each book selected for inclusion. The files are processed to give a consistently clear, crisp image, and the books finished to the high quality standard for which the Press is recognised around the world. The latest print-on-demand technology ensures that the books will remain available indefinitely, and that orders for single or multiple copies can quickly be supplied.

The Cambridge Library Collection brings back to life books of enduring scholarly value (including out-of-copyright works originally issued by other publishers) across a wide range of disciplines in the humanities and social sciences and in science and technology.

Women as Army Surgeons

*Being the History of the
Women's Hospital Corps in Paris,
Wimereux and Endell Street,
September 1914–October 1919*

F LORA M URRAY

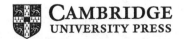
CAMBRIDGE
UNIVERSITY PRESS

CAMBRIDGE
UNIVERSITY PRESS

University Printing House, Cambridge, CB2 8BS, United Kingdom

Published in the United States of America by Cambridge University Press, New York

Cambridge University Press is part of the University of Cambridge.
It furthers the University's mission by disseminating knowledge in the pursuit of
education, learning and research at the highest international levels of excellence.

www.cambridge.org
Information on this title: www.cambridge.org/9781108069854

© in this compilation Cambridge University Press 2014

This edition first published 1920
This digitally printed version 2014

ISBN 978-1-108-06985-4 Paperback

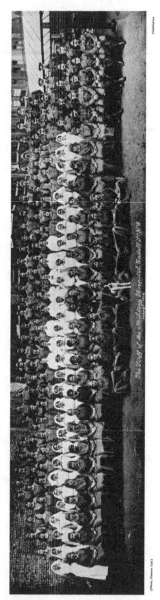

The material originally positioned here is too large for reproduction in this reissue. A PDF can be downloaded from the web address given on page iv of this book, by clicking on 'Resources Available'.

WOMEN AS ARMY SURGEONS

BEING THE HISTORY OF THE WOMEN'S HOSPITAL CORPS IN PARIS, WIMEREUX AND ENDELL STREET

SEPTEMBER 1914—OCTOBER 1919

BY

FLORA MURRAY

C.B.E., M.D., D.P.H.

HODDER AND STOUGHTON
LIMITED   LONDON

TO THE WOMEN'S HOSPITAL CORPS

DEAR FELLOW MEMBERS—This little book has been written for you and for your pleasure.

Your work was too good to be left unrecorded; and though in these pages I have said little in praise, yet if you will read between the lines you will find there a very genuine affection for each one of you, and admiration and pride for your courage and endurance. I ask you to accept *Women as Army Surgeons* in memory of 'Endell Street.'

FLORA MURRAY.

PREFACE

THIS record of the work of the Women's Hospital Corps in France, and especially at the Military Hospital, Endell Street, is a valuable contribution to the literature of the Woman Movement. Dr. Flora Murray and Dr. Garrett Anderson made history at Endell Street. Through their initiative, endeavour, and efficiency they opened the doors to further fields of opportunity for women physicians and surgeons, and not only for medical women, but for all women who are setting out, or have already set out to conquer fresh territory. We owe them a debt of gratitude, the recognition of which will become even more accentuated as the years go on.

It would be difficult to put into words the pride with which the members of the Women's Hospital Corps served their country in the Great War under the only woman Lieutenant-Colonel in the British Army. For this was the rank of Dr. Flora Murray when acting as Doctor-in-Charge at the Military Hospital, Endell Street. The War Office withheld from her both the title and the outward and

visible signs of authority. But the position, with
its responsibilities, pains, and penalties, was hers,
and it is well known how she and the Chief
Surgeon, Dr. Louisa Garrett Anderson, rose to
the demands of the occasion.

It is only on reading these pages that many of
us who worked with them at Endell Street will
realise even partially the difficulties and anxieties
through which they passed during the four years
and more that the Hospital remained open. They
had a double responsibility all through: firstly,
for the lives and welfare of the soldiers entrusted
to their care, and secondly, for the demonstration
of women's efficiency and vindication of the confidence placed in their professional and administrative abilities. If they had failed to satisfy the
Authorities even in the slightest detail, there is
not much doubt but that the charge of the
Hospital would have been handed over to a man,
and that more than one military official would
have had the joy and triumph of saying : ' *There—
I told you so. The women have failed medically
and administratively, and have been unable to maintain discipline.*'

But the opportunity did not occur. The weeks,
the months, the years went on. Thousands of
soldiers poured in and out of that Hospital. A

year after Armistice found it still open. The women had succeeded—not failed, and had set a living example of what trained and disciplined women could do in the service of their country.

Perhaps our C.O. will forgive me for being personal enough to refer to one of her characteristics which was greatly appreciated by all—the trust she reposed in those working under her. You were given your task, your opportunity, your department, and you went ahead with it. It was yours—your own. If you could not do it, you went. If you could, you stayed. She interfered with no details, and harassed you with no unnecessary restrictions. She took it for granted that you were carrying on in the right way and in the right spirit—and judged by results whether it were desirable that you should continue to carry on. In this way you became and remained a living part of the administration. Work and personality alike were benefited, and the young received a baptism of responsibility, destined to influence them favourably for the rest of their lives.

This is surely a great characteristic—and rare.

It is not to be wondered at that the success of this Military Hospital, officered, staffed, and run entirely by women, became a source of immense

satisfaction and pride to all women, but more
especially to those who had taken an active part
in the struggle for the Suffrage, and had shared,
with Dr. Flora Murray and Dr. Garrett Anderson,
the ups and downs, the hopes and fears, the disappointments, disillusions, and encouragements,
and all the stress and strain of a long-drawn-out
political campaign. To these, Endell Street represented work for the country and work for the
woman movement combined, and to the members
of the Women's Hospital Corps itself it meant, in
addition, a double chance of service, a double devotion, a double inspiration, a double reason for
carrying on with undiminished enthusiasm and
faithfulness to the end.

                    BEATRICE HARRADEN.

4th August 1920.

CONTENTS

PART I

THE WOMEN'S HOSPITAL CORPS IN PARIS AND WIMEREUX

ILLUSTRATIONS

PART I

THE WOMEN'S HOSPITAL CORPS
IN PARIS AND WIMEREUX

CHAPTER I

ORGANISATION OF THE WOMEN'S HOSPITAL CORPS

In August 1914 it was a popular idea that war was man's business and that everything and every one else should stand aside and let men act. But there were many persons who failed to endorse this view and who held that, though men may have been responsible for the war, the business of it concerned men and women equally. Far from standing aside and leaving men to act alone, every woman in the land accepted her duty and her responsibility, and recognised at once that if the war was to be won it must be won by the whole nation, and by the common effort of all her children.

The long years of struggle for the Enfranchisement of Women which had preceded the outbreak of war had done much to educate women in citizenship and in public duty. The militant movement had taught them discipline and organisation; it had shown them new possibilities in themselves, and had inspired them with confidence

3

in each other. In face of the greater militancy
of men, the Suffragists called a truce, and set
their adherents free for service in government
departments, in factories and in hospitals. Work-
rooms were opened, day-nurseries established and
surgical supply depots commenced their useful
labours.

Women who had been trained in medicine and
in surgery knew instinctively that the time had
come when great and novel demands would be
made upon them, and that a hitherto unlooked-
for occasion for service was at their feet. It was
inconceivable that in a war of such magnitude
women doctors should not join in the care of the
sick and wounded, but it was obvious that prejudice would stand in their way. Their training
and their sympathies fitted them for such
work ; they knew and could trust their own
capacity ; but they had yet to make their
opportunity.

Amongst others, Dr. Louisa Garrett Anderson
and Dr. Flora Murray were determined that
medical women desiring to give their services to
the nation should not be excluded from military
work and from the great professional opportunities
naturally arising from it. An opening, therefore,
had to be found for them. As militant suffragists

they had had dealings with the Home Office, and
had gained an insight into the cherished prejudices and stereotyped outlook of officials. One
government department is very like another, and
to have approached the War Office at that time
would only have meant to court a rebuff. But
it was common knowledge that the French Army
was inadequately supplied with surgeons and
hospitals ; and they turned their attention where
the need was great.

On the 12th of August these two doctors called
at the French Embassy and were received by one
of the secretaries in an absolutely airless room.
The atmosphere was enhanced by red damask
wall hangings and upholstery, and by an aroma
of stale cigar smoke. In somewhat rusty French
they laid before him an offer to raise and equip a
surgical unit for service in France. The secretary
may have been rather mystified as to their intentions ; for medical women were off his horizon.
Very likely he never realised that they themselves
intended to go to the aid of the French wounded ;
but he affirmed again and again the real need of
France for medical and surgical aid, for stores of
all kinds and for English nurses. He begged
' Mesdames ' to call upon the President of the
French Red Cross in London and discuss the matter

with her, and, tendering with the utmost courtesy a card of introduction, he directed them to her house.

Madame Brasier de Thuy was the President of the branch of the French Red Cross known as ' L'Union des Femmes de France.' The title of her Society was attractive, and she herself combined great charm of manner with a pleasing personality. Although she was oppressed with anxiety for the safety of France and the welfare of her relations, she was working hard to raise money and necessaries for the French Red Cross.

She had few fellow-workers and no organisation to help her, and both she and Monsieur Brasier de Thuy often wrote and toiled far into the night. She received with great cordiality the offer of a fully equipped surgical unit, comprised of women doctors and trained nurses. Surgeons were a godsend and English nurses an indescribable boon. No difficulties were raised; and the offer was transmitted to the headquarters of her Society in Paris. Within a week, a formal acceptance from Paris reached Dr. Garrett Anderson, accompanied by a request that the unit might be organised at once and be ready, if required, to start on the 1st of September.

There remained exactly twelve days of August
in which to raise the funds required, find a staff
and purchase the equipment and all the stores
which would be needed.

The appeal for money was made privately and
met with a prompt and generous response. Mrs.
Garrett Anderson, M.D., Mrs. Granger and Sir
Alan Anderson led the way with large donations.
Miss S. A. Turle, Miss Janie Allan and other
women interested in women's work sent liberal
help. Letters of encouragement and further subscriptions poured in, and within a fortnight the
sum of £2000 was placed to the credit of the
Women's Hospital Corps, which was the name
decided upon for the unit.

This amount was enough to purchase the
equipment, defray the preliminary expenses and
leave a working balance in hand.

At that time the authorities in Paris had not
decided where the Corps was to be located; it
was thought that it might be established in a
château near Belfort, where it would have to be
self-dependent; and this possibility had to be
taken into account when making purchases.
Comprehensive lists of drugs, stores and hospital
equipment were drawn up with a view to all
emergencies. Many kinds of serum were included,

with cases of invalid foods and chloroform, chests of tea, clothing, blankets, camp bedsteads, enamel ware and a full set of surgical instruments. Altogether, £1000 was spent on the equipment, which afterwards proved to be adequate for the needs of both the hospitals managed by the Corps.

Offers of service were gladly accepted from Dr. Gertrude Gazdar, Dr. Hazel Cuthbert and Dr. Grace Judge. Many applications were considered from nurses and from girls anxious to go out as supernumeraries or orderlies; and the staff was rapidly completed. It was decided to include a few male nurses, and in order to find suitable men recourse was had to the St. John's Ambulance Association, at St. John's Gate, Clerkenwell.

In these early days every public office probably presented an air of chaos, and 'The Gate' was no exception. In the central hall a swarm of people circulated without ceasing through a maze of chairs and tables; loud crashes of falling furniture, due to the entanglement of umbrellas and draperies, punctuated the incessant conversations. Every one was friendly, anxious to help and willing to work, but the confusion and noise of voices had a bewildering effect.

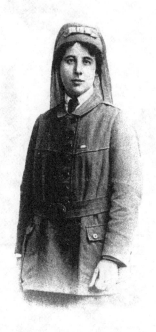

ORDERLY HODGSON IN THE UNIFORM
OF THE WOMEN'S HOSPITAL CORPS

(Page 10)

(Photo, Stuart)

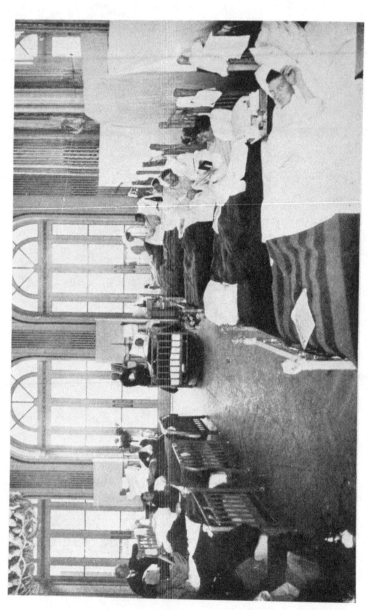

A WARD IN THE HÔTEL CLARIDGE

(Page 11)

In the smaller rooms some kind of departmental order was growing. With real kindness, the authorities gave advice and assistance, and one of the officials put the doctors into touch with two first-class male nurses, who proved most valuable assistants.

The place was full of rumours and of special information brought over by its Commissioners about military matters and German atrocities. All the head officials appeared to have different opinions and to come to different decisions, and one old gentleman, who held a high office, kept saying, ' Kitchener will never let you cross, you know. Does Kitchener know you are going ? He won't let any one cross.'

' The Gate ' distrusted the French Red Cross, and was quite sure that if anything was left for it to do it would be muddled ; and the French Red Cross could not understand why ' The Gate ' should offer to arrange about passports and baggage, since it was quite able to do all that itself. As a matter of fact, the arrangements for the transport of baggage were made, and most excellently made, by Monsieur Brasier de Thuy.

The packing was done by Messrs. John Barker & Co., of Kensington, a firm which also supplied

a great part of the equipment. When the bales
and boxes were complete, they were piled in the
street outside their premises and made an imposing
array. There were more than a hundred packages
—many large Red Cross cases with padlocks, all
labelled and painted with 'Croix Rouge Fran-
çaise' and 'Women's Hospital Corps,' with lists
of their contents noted on them and the address.
Piled on the top of them were enormous bales of
wool and blankets, pillows and clothing. The
display attracted crowds of interested spectators
as it lay under the awnings, and members of the
Corps who saw it thrilled with anticipation and
eagerness.

The uniform of the Corps had been chosen
carefully. It consisted of a short skirt with a
loose, well-buttoned-up tunic, and was made of
covert coating of a greenish-grey colour. The
material was light and durable, and stood wear
and weather well. The medical officers had red
shoulder straps with the Corps initials, 'W.H.C.,'
worked on them in white, and the orderlies had
white collars and shoulder straps with red letters.
The white was not serviceable, and at a later date
blue was substituted for it. Small cloth hats
with veils and overcoats to match made a very
comfortable and useful outfit.

That uniform was a passport which admitted the women who wore it to offices, bureaus, stations, canteens, wherever their work took them. It was equally correct in hospitals, in ambulances, in the streets of Paris and among troops. In some magic way it opened doors and hearts and pockets.

The Parisians murmured, ' C'est chic, ça ! '

The senior British officer asked, ' Who designed your uniform ? '

And the subaltern said, ' Where did you get that jolly kit ? '

Feminine, graceful, business-like, it was invaluable as an introduction to the character of the Corps.

Before leaving England, it was necessary to appoint a representative in London to receive gifts and to send over these and any extra things which might be wanted. Dr. Louisa Woodcock undertook this work, and found that it was no sinecure. For as soon as the work of the hospital in Paris became known at home, her correspondence increased by leaps and bounds and her house was crowded with sacks and parcels coming from all parts of the country.

Her interest in the formation of the unit was only equalled by that of Mrs. Garrett Anderson, the pioneer woman doctor, who, though eighty years of age, came up to London in order that she might hear all the details at first hand.

' If you go,' she said, ' and if you succeed, you will put your cause forward a hundred years.'

CHAPTER II

ARRIVAL IN PARIS

THE authorities in Paris did not require the unit to travel until later than the date originally suggested. It was September before they decided that it should be located in Paris and should open a hospital in the Hôtel Claridge, which had been placed at the disposal of the French Red Cross.

On Tuesday the 14th of September 1914 the Women's Hospital Corps left Victoria for Paris. The heavy baggage had gone the day before, and was to be forwarded on the boat by which the party would travel. Empty trucks were to await it on the other side, and these were to be attached to the Paris train.

A personal friend among the traffic managers reserved a saloon for the travellers and procured them the great privilege of having friends on the platform to see them off. This was immensely appreciated, and many well-wishers gathered round them, offering greetings and tokens of affection

in the form of flowers and fruits. Madame
Brasier de Thuy and her husband, accompanied
by several French ladies, were there. Mrs. Granger came with her arms full of grapes. Many
women doctors, well-known suffragists, journalists and photographers joined the little crowd.
Relatives brought roses and chocolates, and ladies
with sons in France asked that letters and parcels
might be conveyed to them.

A little apart, Mrs. Garrett Anderson, a dignified
figure, old and rather bent, stood quietly observing
the bustle and handshaking. One wondered of
what she was thinking as she contemplated this
development of the work she had begun. Her
eyes were tender and wistful as she watched her
daughter in uniform directing the party and
calling the roll of the Corps. A friend beside her
said :

' Are you not proud, Mrs. Anderson ? '

The light of battle—of old battles fought long
ago—came into her face as she raised her head
and surveyed the scene.

' Yes,' she answered. ' Twenty years younger,
I would have taken them myself.'

Late that afternoon the boat steamed into
Dieppe, past the long low lines of the Quay,

outlined by silent, watching people. As the women in uniform followed one by one down the gangway, the groups of sailors and porters gazed at them with grave attention. The English Consul had come to meet them, and wished that they were staying in Dieppe ; for the hospitals were crowded with wounded and there were not enough helpers. The agent, M. Guérin, was there too, with his complement of empty trucks for the baggage, which, it now transpired, had not been put on the boat. The perjured purser, who had given assurances that all was well, stood ashamed ; but M. Guérin, claiming him as a great friend of his son, demanded that he should use his best endeavours to expedite the missing luggage. Leaving them to arrange the matter between them, the women followed the Consul to the Douane.

A picturesque old French lady in a chenille cap asked no questions but made marks with a stubby bit of chalk on the hand-baggage ; an excitable British Red Cross lady explained that nothing was any good here. ' The red tape was awful— all the arrangements had broken down. The sepsis was appalling. The town was full of Germans whose legs and arms had been cut off and who were being sent to Havre next day like that ! ! '

And so talking the party came to the station, and travelling like soldiers, 'sans billets,' on account of their uniform, they were hustled into the train, which jolted slowly away.

The last part of the journey was very slow, and Paris was not reached till ten o'clock at night. From Pontoise onwards the train was held up at every little station, and gentlemen in blue blouses came to the carriage windows asking with immense interest who the travellers were and where they were going, or volunteering amazing information on military matters, and as it grew dark indicating lights which they called patrolling aeroplanes or signals or searchlights.

The Gare du Nord was dimly lit and there were no porters on the platform, but a representative of the French Red Cross met the train with the information that rooms were reserved in the Station Hotel. He watched with silent astonishment while Orderly Campbell and Orderly Hodgson commandeered a large luggage trolley and, having loaded it with all the bags and wraps, proceeded to trundle it out of the station. Then drawing a deep breath, he led the way through the darkness to the hotel. The station entrance to it was locked; the lifts were not working; the *cuisinier* was mobilised. There could be no supper.

Impossible even to make a *chocolat.* But there were bedrooms on the third floor, and the ladies might go up and take their choice. So, shouldering the bags, they mounted the half-lit staircase, found a whole corridor of rooms at their disposal, and settled down cheerfully to picnic out of the still well-stocked luncheon baskets.

The following morning the President of the French Red Cross, Madame Pérouse, called at the Hôtel to discuss matters with Dr. Louisa Garrett Anderson and Dr. Flora Murray. She was a charming old lady, gentle and unaccustomed to office work. She was confused by the multiple claims made upon her, and oppressed by the burden of work, which was far beyond her strength and her powers.

Speaking no language but her own, without a stenographer or typewriter, and supported by officials who were all advanced in years, her difficulties must have been very great, and no one could blame her if she was not entirely successful. There was friction to contend with between the three branches of the Red Cross, which caused overlapping instead of co-ordination of effort ; and each and every section had obstruction to meet from the Army Medical Department, the military authorities and the Military Governor

B

of Paris. Thus, if the Society seemed slow in
its decisions and uncertain in its action, there
were extenuating circumstances ; and the number of old people at the head of affairs could
not fail to be a drawback. For has it not
been written : ' Men of age object too much,
consult too long, adventure too little, repent too
soon, and seldom drive business home to the full
period ' ?

Madame Pérouse was accompanied by an
English doctor, who was attached to another
voluntary hospital. He gave a lurid account
of the French Army, its hospitals and the state
of its wounded as he saw them, including in his
remarks advice against trusting the French Red
Cross or anything else that was French. While
he talked to Dr. Garrett Anderson, Dr. Murray
came to an understanding with Madame Pérouse.
Realising that the old lady really did not know
what she wanted them to do and had no instructions to give, she proposed that they should go
with her to the Hôtel Claridge and inform themselves as to the possibilities of that building.

The Hôtel Claridge was a large modern cara-
vanserai on the Champs Élysées. As the builders
had only just completed their work, the walls
were hardly dry, and the floors were covered with

débris. The whitening had not been cleaned off the windows, and men were still working at the electric light and in the boiler house. On the ground floor a series of large salons and dining-rooms opened out of one another. They had been designed so that no ray of sunlight ever entered them! But they were structurally capable of making good wards for a hundred patients. Luxurious and comfortably furnished bedrooms on the first floor offered accommodation for the staff, and large stores of new beds and expensive blankets were available. The building was intersected by long gloomy corridors, each one laid with an elaborate tesselated pavement and decorated with enormous mirrors. The *chauffage* had not yet been persuaded to act, and the atmosphere was cold and damp ; but there were many conveniences in the shape of gas ovens and sinks as well as service-rooms—a fact which made the Hôtel a suitable place for a hospital.

The French Red Cross had already accepted the services of a Red Cross commandant and a small party of English nurses, and had quartered them in the Hôtel. Madame Pérouse proposed to attach them to the staff of the Women's Hospital Corps and to let them work under the direction of the doctors. In the kitchen a chef had been installed, with some Belgian women to assist him, and the rest of the establishment included M. Perrin, the engineer, and M. André, the concierge, with his wife and family.

It was obvious that the Unit ought to move in at once and begin to get the wards into order. Meanwhile, there were certain formalities to be observed. The members of the staff had to be registered with the police ; cards of identity had to be issued for each one of them ; photographs were needed to complete these ; and arm brassards with cryptic figures must be procured from the offices of the French Red Cross in the rue de Thann.

The Red Cross offices were the scene of great activity. In one large room numbers of ladies were engaged in writing examination papers which would qualify them as nurses after an intensive fifteen days' course of study. They were ' très bien mises,' and the first lecture of the course gave careful instructions for the care of the hands and complexion, and included recipes for the preparation of *pommades* and other cosmetics ! In an adjacent room ladies in white robes were winding bandages ; and an office upstairs was tenanted by two gentlemen who occupied the position of *directeurs*.

The senior of these two was M. le Docteur M——, a man of a highly irritable nature which made him a terror to the Red Cross ladies. ' Pour rien du tout,' they whispered, his long grey hair would stand on end, his pendulous cheeks quiver and his corpulent person be convulsed ; then, with threatening finger and bitter gibes, he would drive them from his presence. His method of conducting affairs was unintelligible to British people ; and seeing how obstructive and perverse he was, it was a marvel that his staff accomplished anything. Dr. Garrett Anderson and Dr. Flora Murray, having stated their requirements to a secretary, were asked to sit down while he made out some papers for them, and from two chairs against the wall they had leisure to make their observations. With deep interest they heard a senior clerk try to obtain a decision from M. le Docteur and his white-haired, sleepy colleague as to the situation of ' L'Hôpital Base des Alliés.' Both directors were deaf, and he had to read the letter in question in a loud voice. The letter was ten days old, and the clerk urged this as a reason for deciding that afternoon.

' Il y a déjà dix jours,' he pleaded.

' Et s'il y avait vingt jours ! ' roared M. le Docteur ; and suddenly subsided as he became aware of the interested spectators against the wall.

The clerk tried another line, produced a map and made further suggestions; but the older gentleman was tired of the matter. He turned his back on his colleague—still growling over the map—and concentrated his attention upon ' ces dames anglaises.'

The papers being ready, the secretary directed them to another office where brassards might be obtained. Here a lady, with great volubility and in most rapid French, explained her intricate reasons for not giving them any ! And as they did not much mind whether they had them or not, they bade her a friendly farewell and left the premises. Just outside they met M. Falcouz and laid the foundation of a pleasant little friendship. With his white hair ' en brosse ' and his little tufted beard, he presented a sufficiently un-English and interesting appearance. It was his habit always to dress in black and to wear a black satin tie and gloves two sizes too large for him. He was the Red Cross Treasurer, and as beseemed his office, he beamed on the doctors and fell to discussing money matters.

' Have you money ? How have you raised it ? ' he asked.

On hearing how the money had been found, he exclaimed :

' Épatant.'

And then added :

' In France it would not be possible, mesdames. Nobody would be trusted with such a sum ! '

CHAPTER III

THE HOSPITAL IN THE HÔTEL CLARIDGE IS OPENED

THE second morning in Paris found the Corps busily engaged at the Hôtel Claridge. There was a great deal of cleaning to do and many arrangements to make before the place would be habitable. In the centre of the building was a handsome paved hall with a many-coloured marble table and enormous glass chandeliers. Out of this four good-sized salons opened, and it was in these that wards were first arranged.

The salons were only divided from one another by plate glass; and some degree of privacy is necessary for a ward. Doctors and nurses alike put on aprons and rolled up their sleeves, and while some cleaned the whitening off the glass, the others pasted the lower part over with white paper. With help from the Belgian refugees, who were lodged on the seventh story, the floors were cleaned and polished, beds were put up and order began to be evolved.

The ladies' cloakroom, with its pavement, its

24

hot-water supply and basins, was converted into the operating theatre. A gas steriliser and a powerful electric light were fixed in it. Though small, it proved serviceable and well equipped.

The cleaning was sufficiently advanced to allow of the Corps moving into its quarters on the first floor next day, and they spent the morning carrying bedding and furniture down to the wards. These at once began to have a professional look, and by concentrating on two wards they were successful in getting fifty beds prepared for patients by the evening.

The work of preparation was at its height when a doctor from the American hospital walked in. Upon the outbreak of the war, the American colony in Paris had organised their fine hospital in the Lycée at Neuilly and had established a fleet of ambulances. Their ambulances enabled them to carry hundreds of men from the fighting line in to Paris. Both French and British wounded were in terrible straits ; for there was no organised motor transport service, and the Armies depended on the railways for the removal of the sick and injured. The long delays and the conditions under which the men lay whilst waiting for removal were fatal, and the American service was the means of saving numbers of lives.

When trains were available the wounded were packed into them and despatched to distant places in the interior. As they passed Paris, those who were so severely wounded that they were unlikely to survive a long journey were left at the stations on the Circle Railway round the city. There they would lie on straw or sacks, waiting for friendly ambulances to come out and bring them in.

In those first weeks there was no system of communication between the hospitals and the stations ; the French ambulances were small and bad, and the British had none available for Paris. The matter depended largely upon individual effort, and the ambulances of the American and other voluntary hospitals played a devoted and humanitarian part.

The doctor from Neuilly was in charge of the ambulance service. The American hospital was already very full of French and British, but, in response to a message which he had received, he was sending out his cars that day, and he hoped that there might be beds ready for some of the cases at ' Claridge's.'

' How many can you take ? ' he asked.

' We can take twenty-four this afternoon and another twenty-six to-night,' replied Dr. Murray, well knowing that the baggage was still at the station, and conscious of the expression on the faces of those who heard her.

' Good ! Will you take officers ? ' he said.

' Yes. We have a ward for officers,' she answered, remembering for the first time that officers get wounded as well as men, and that no special pyjamas or cambric handkerchiefs had been included in the equipment !

' Well, I shall bring officers,' he said ; ' British ladies are the right people to look after British officers.' And remarking that he only brought in severe cases, and that they would all need immediate operations, he left the staff to face the inadequacy of their preparations from the officer's point of view.

' At any rate, they 'll have lovely beds, if nothing else,' Orderly Campbell remarked, with a reassuring laugh.

Fortunately, a notice had come from the Railway Company that morning to say that the baggage was at the station, and Orderly Hodgson had started early to retrieve it. She spent hours dealing with the intricate formalities required by the Company and finding transport for the baggage ; but she stuck to it resolutely, and drove in triumph to the door with it a few minutes before the first ambulance full of wounded arrived. The stretchers and the packing cases were carried into the hall side by side, and while the nurses and surgeons cared for the patients, the orderlies unpacked the equipment.

As those first stretchers with their weary burdens were carried in, a thrill of pity and dismay ran through the women who saw them. The mud-stained khaki and the unshaven faces spoke to them no less than the wounded limbs and shattered nerves. Here, for the first time, they touched the wastage and the desolation of war. In every wounded man they saw some other woman's husband or son, and the thought of those other women made a double claim on their energy and sympathy. The battered, inarticulate, suffering men who lay there needed service, and they braced themselves for the work before them.

Organisation developed automatically : nurses for night duty were sent to rest ; the theatre sister began to sterilise ; chloroform, instruments, drugs and dressings were produced and distributed.

Late in the afternoon a message from the Chief Surgeon was brought from the wards :

' Dr. Anderson wishes to know if the theatre is ready and if she can operate to-night.'

' It is ready now,' was the answer.

And the surgeons operated till a late hour that night.

The hospital was a smooth-running concern by the end of the week. Nurses and patients had settled down in the wards ; work in the operating theatre was going well ; and though it was far from perfect in all its details, the comfort of the officers and men was assured, and their contentment and satisfaction with their surroundings were very pleasant to see.

CHAPTER IV

FIRST DAYS IN PARIS

THE streets of Paris were strangely altered and unfamiliar, with closed shops and whole blocks of houses empty and shuttered. The Government was at Bordeaux, and the Louvre and all places of amusement were shut. Only the churches were crowded, and from their dark interiors the side altars shone out, brilliantly lighted and surrounded by women and children on their knees. Day by day they trooped past the altars, lighting the candles and offering their prayers; and day by day the casualty lists grew longer and the number of crêpe veils in the streets increased.

Life was not easy for the women of Paris, but they bore themselves with great dignity and courage. Their attitude was calm and reticent; they took over men's posts in the shops and work-rooms, or on the trams and railways, as a matter of course, and carried out their duties with quiet efficiency.

The uniform of the Women's Hospital Corps

soon became known, and secured a cordial reception for its members in the bureaux and offices which they had to visit, as well as on the boulevards. Strangers would offer them gifts of socks and mittens. Old ladies, with tears running down their cheeks, would lift their outer skirts and rummage in the *poche intérieur* to bestow a few francs with a blessing upon them. An Englishman, choking with emotion, put two sovereigns into a doctor's hand as she passed him on the stairs of the Hôtel. Shopkeepers asked about 'les blessés' and sent presents of sweets and biscuits. The greengrocer added an extra cauliflower to the purchase ! Flower-women ran after them and pressed bunches of roses into their hands.

At the entrance of the Hôtel when ambulances were unloading, elderly men in silk hats and black kid gloves would crowd round and offer to carry the stretchers, or would follow the bearers inside, with the kit—often a very dirty kit—in their arms. The sight of the suffering moved them so that they turned aside and wept. They brought violets and roses and cigarettes for the men. They stood outside the doors to listen to them singing, and they wrung the hands of the doctors silently and went out. The people were deeply moved, but not cast down. They had settled

---

down to war, and even then they were confident of victory, since the English were with them.

The cordiality of the people, the general sympathy and the inspiration of a common cause, combined with the beauty of Paris and the charm of the autumn weather to make these days a wonderful memory.

The organisation of the hospital proceeded rapidly, and the amount of heavy surgery and acute sepsis which came in taxed the energy and resources of the surgical staff. Dr. Garrett Anderson acted as chief surgeon and Dr. Gazdar took charge of the officers' ward. Other workers fell into their places and a sort of routine was gradually evolved. The duties of administrator, or *Médecin-en-Chef*, fell to Dr. Flora Murray, and when she was not issuing stores or counting linen, she would be receiving the countless visitors who came to see the wards.

The French Red Cross wished the hospital to have a *directeur*, and for this purpose they attached to it M. Aubry, a French gentleman who was at leisure during the closure of the stock exchange. He spoke French only, and his duties as director were purely nominal. He was considerate and genial, and the staff became very fond of him.

He had a son in the Dragoons of whom he was immensely proud ; and the arrival of a grandson, or *petit dragon*, was a great social event in which every one shared. He seemed to spend several hours a day chatting with any one who had time to listen to him, and occasionally he joined the mess for tea. He helped the work of the hospital greatly by bringing in one of his clerks, M. Gohin, to take charge of the registers and returns.

The French Army required an immense number of returns to be made. These had to be rendered in the form of a nominal roll, on the fifth day, the tenth day, and the twenty-fifth day of each man's stay in hospital. As the men did not all come in on the same day, the return of the yellow or blue or white cards—as the case might be—was never-ending. The British made it simpler, for one nominal roll went every week to the War Office and a copy of it to the R.A.M.C. authorities in Paris.

M. Gohin was unfit for military service, but he certainly made good by the skill with which he managed a very complicated and tiresome piece of clerical work.

Sundry other youthful clerks also came from M. Aubry's office to assist in the wards, and his

C

concierge, M. Roget, took the hospital under his wing. M. Roget had been with M. Aubry for a great many years, and he loved and admired him dearly. His affection frequently prompted him to discuss the appearance and ways of his master when he was 'en colère.' At such times he was said to resemble a wild beast, and no one could calm him except Roget. Every morning, in a white pinafore, with a little watering-pot in his hand, M. Roget would perambulate the central hall, covering the pavement with moist curls and twists. Then he would throw a little sawdust about and leave it for some one else to sweep. He was a great man for rumours, and when he was not giving details of his anatomy and his pathological condition, he would have mysterious tales of a hundred trains that had gone from Paris to the Front to bring in German prisoners ; of spies and plots within the walls of Paris ; or of great military events which were to end the war in six weeks.

The management of the Hôtel itself was in the hands of M. Casanova, who acted as *directeur* under the Company which had built and owned it. He was short and stout, with a flowing black beard, and soft, well-manicured little hands, very courteous and agreeable, prolific of promises, which for some reason never seemed to be fulfilled. He was moved to the very depths of his self-indulgent soul by the war and the proximity of suffering and wounded men. He would descend at night in his pyjamas if he heard a convoy coming in, and penetrate to the wards to see what was going on, and to offer help. Though not in the best of health, he would fetch hot water or lift weights. He would reach out a trembling hand to hold things, while he wiped his eyes with the other. His sympathy and distress, combined with a desire to kiss the busy hands of the doctors, made him a touching figure.

In his train were always strange ladies, wrapped in blankets, who followed him and peeped round the doors. His rooms were luxurious. His menu was *spécial*. But he roused himself to serve and to help with all sincerity. Unfortunately, his relations with M. Aubry became somewhat strained at a later stage, for he had a passionate temperament. There were wont to be terrible domestic uproars below stairs. M. Casanova's method of administering justice was to declare that some one was *coupable* of breaking into the wine-cellars, eating too much butter or causing the cheese to disappear. He accused everybody, and everybody asserted his innocence; so he said they must draw lots as to which of them must be *chassés*. The lot fell on four Belgian girls who hung about the place and did *services*; at this the rest of the staff was up in arms, and M. Perrin, the engineer, said, if they were *chassées*, he also would be *chassé*; and in a perfect storm of rage and recrimination it was decided that every one was to be *chassés*. M. Perrin disappeared. The apparatus for the supply of hot water and heating ran down in his absence, and the Belgian girls wailed that they were being cast upon the streets.

The *Médecin-en-Chef* waited upon M. Casanova in the interest of the girls. He presented her with twelve cakes of soap and some scent:

' As a testimony of my admiration for your courage and nobility,' he said.

And, kissing her hand, he added:

' The members of *l'équipe* under your distinguished direction, madame, are models of virtue and devotion; but there are others of whom one can say nothing but evil.'

His mood, however, softened, and in the morning it was understood that no one was to leave, and, to the relief of all concerned, M. Perrin returned and resumed his duties.

The officials of the French Red Cross were delighted with the rapid way in which the hospital had got to work, and took a great interest in all that was being done there. Not infrequently Madame Pérouse, accompanied by M. Falcouz, would arrive to pay a visit at eight o'clock in the morning. The first greetings over, she would suggest going to greet the officers—'prendre de leurs nouvelles,' so she put it. At that hour the ward work was in full swing, and any one who has had experience of nurses knows how the Sister feels when visitors arrive before she is ready. British officers, too, prefer to have time to break-fast and shave before being inspected. But the dear old people were oblivious of their embarrass-ment and entered the ward with genial ' Bon-jours.' They asked the major how he was and he replied, with grave courtesy, ' Merci, madame ; merci, monsieur.' They asked the others one by one if they spoke French, and they replied sever-ally, ' Pas beaucoup,' or ' Un petit peu.' And so, bowing and gracious, they passed on their tour of inspection.

In those days very few officers seemed able to speak French, and intercourse with their French brothers-at-arms in neighbouring beds was in-conveniently restricted. Referring to the lan-

guage, one of them said, ' The insuperable difficulty of this campaign is the language — it 's
unspeakable ! ' And some of the doctors echoed
his opinion heartily.

Left alone on duty one night, a surgeon wished
to talk to a wounded French officer and was
obliged to ask for the assistance as interpreter
of a nurse who had a reputation as a linguist.

' Ask him,' said the surgeon, ' if he has a pain
in his stomach.'

The nurse bent over the bed and put the question :

' Monsieur, avez-vous du pain dans l'estomac ? '

The poor man had been shot through the body
and was on a water diet. He indignantly repudi-
ated the suggestion, assuring her that he had only
taken what the surgeon had ordered for him and
that under no circumstances would he do otherwise.

Both French and British officers were acutely
shocked by the horrors through which they had
passed, and most of them suffered from a painful
reaction when the strain was relaxed. At first
they could not rest in hospital, and their nights
were haunted by terrible memories and anxious
thoughts. One of them never told what he had
seen, but night after night he covered his face
with his uninjured hand and moaned :

' The children.   Oh ! the children ! '

He had left children of his own at home ; and the sufferings of the little Belgians gave him no rest.

Older men were harassed and worn by anxiety, and distressed by the difficulty and precarious position of the allied Armies. The younger ones spoke of how ' the British were hanging on with their eyelids ' ; or how the French were supposed to be ' making a flank attack and were lost.' Some in their depression feared defeat ; others broke down with exhaustion and reaction.

To all of them, officers and men alike, hospital was a haven of peace and security. It was heavenly to lie in clean beds, to be cared for by Englishwomen, to be rid of regimental discipline and for the moment of responsibility too. The severity of their wounds, the operations, the pain were minor matters ; for the time being they had found comfort and rest. Probably none of them had been in contact with women doctors before ; but that did not make any difference. They trusted the women as they would have trusted men—passing the bullets which had been extracted from their persons from bed to bed and pronouncing the surgeon to be ' wonderfully clever ! ' The more convalescent patients visited the men who had undergone serious operations in the wards and cheered them with reminders that they were not ' in the hands of the R.A.M.C.' Their enthusiasm for the hospital was delightful and encouraging. When they got well and went away, it was like seeing boys go back to school.

The condition of the men was, if possible, worse than that of the officers. They had lain in queer wayside stations, waiting for trains, or on straw in stables and churches, hoping for transport. At Villeneuve, on the Paris railway circle, there was a goods shed with straw on the ground, in which officers lay at one end and men at the other. An R.A.M.C. doctor and a few men did what they could for them, and when the ambulances came out from Paris, the worst were picked out ; but, for the rest, the weary waiting for a train continued. At Creil, forty miles from Paris, the accommodation was an open shed filled with straw. French and British lay huddled in groups, some covered by blankets, others by dirty sacks. A doctor of the French Army, very dapper in his red and blue plush cap, sorted them into trains, when any trains came. Several French soldiers stirred a mess of *potage* with a dirty stick. But of dressings or nursing there was no sign. Patiently and uncomplainingly these sufferers waited, often fifteen, twenty-four or more hours, while the rain poured down on the roof of their shed, and the wind swept drearily through the station.

At last, septic and wasted by fever, they were jolted by the ambulances over the ill-paved roads to Paris and hospital. Lieut. Lowe, whose only chance lay in getting into hospital without further delay, was brought down from Compiègne on a stretcher laid across an ordinary motor-car and held in position by an American doctor and a man with one hand. His thigh was badly fractured and very imperfectly supported ; but with the help of morphia he endured the journey. From the first there was little hope of his recovery, but he lingered for some weeks, during which his sister was able to be with him, lavishing care and tenderness upon him to their mutual comfort.

The men were dirty and half-fed ; many had not had a change of clothes or socks since they left England ; but they were absolutely uncomplaining and began at once to appreciate their hospital surroundings. Women doctors were a novelty which served to enhance the importance and the grandeur of the gilded and marble halls in which they found themselves. ' The doctors is ladies,' they wrote in their letters home ; and to the visitor who asked : ' Is it really true that you

have no men doctors here ? ' the reply was :
' And what will we be wanting men doctors for,
sir ? '

They found comfort in the presence of women
and repose in the care lavished upon them, and
with the philosophy of the soldier they let it
rest there.

CHAPTER V

A VISIT TO BRAISNE, AND AN INSPECTION

GOOD supplies of clothing and hospital comforts found their way to ' Claridge's ' from the many work-parties which had been started in England. Socks and gloves came in sacks from Oban, Edinburgh and Aberdeen ; pillow-cases and shirts from Annan ; belts and bandages from Stoke ; parcels were sent from Cardiff and Bristol ; and hot-water bottles, bed socks and many other welcome gifts arrived from other places. The Corps had plenty of socks and shirts to send to the outlying stations through which troops passed, or to the places where collections of wounded were known to be lying. French soldiers, too, learned that there were socks to be had, and many of them came to the Hôtel to ask for a pair. They emphasised their need by drawing rubbed and bruised feet, bound in rags, from their army boots, lamenting that the smallness of their pay would not run to socks. With a nice pair, knitted by some one in Scotland, and a little box of ointment they went out beaming.

Two Paris friends, Mlle Block and Miss Grey, gave the hospital very real assistance by providing two ambulances and placing them at the disposal of the medical staff. They were both of them splendid drivers, and they did many a hard day's work, and thought no pains too great, no journey too long, that gave some wounded man a chance of recovery.

When the R.A.M.C. officer at Braisne telephoned to ask for ' shirts and anything else you can send,' a car with all sorts of necessary articles was got ready. A bundle of shirts, a sack of socks, a case of invalid foods and a large bag of dressings were piled in. All the English papers which could be collected and a supply of Woodbines and some books were added, for distribution to the British troops who were always found on the roads or resting in the villages ; and the whole was despatched in the care of the Chief Surgeon early one morning in September.

The country was beautiful in the autumn sunlight. It looked peaceful too, as her car followed the long straight roads. But there were shallow trenches by the roadside and barricades, with sentries at intervals, which spoke of war. English

soldiers were met, who cheerfully relieved her of
the papers and books, and appreciated the Woodbines and the matches ; or asked for news from
home, and gave her letters to post in Paris. At
every village the *permis* and the contents of the
car were examined, and when Paris was left
behind, troops were seen moving in large numbers.
Wherever the car stopped, villagers crowded round
it, eager to tell ' l'Anglaise ' how the ' Uhlans '
had come so far : how they had fired the houses
and emptied the cellars, and how they had been
driven out, and how terrible war was. The smoke
of the German guns firing on Soissons was visible
as the driver turned off towards Braisne.

The little town, which looked destitute and
untidy, lay in a hollow with bare hills all round it,
and Dr. Garrett Anderson, as she drove down the
main street, could tell by the stench in which
buildings the wounded lay. She was met by the
R.A.M.C. officer, who asked her to come to headquarters, and took her to a dilapidated little
house in which the officers had their mess. She
followed her guide through the house into a small
backyard where three officers were sitting round
a wooden table eating bread and cheese. The
colonel said he had not much time, but he would
like her to sit down and talk to him while he ate.

And a wooden stool was found for her. The air of the place was close and fetid, the flies buzzed over the food, and the men looked careworn and lined. The squalor and discomfort were oppressive, and she was glad when the meal was finished and she could go out into the street with the R.A.M.C. officer, who stayed closely by her. The car was unloaded, and when he saw what she had brought his voice shook as he thanked her. He was young, and the strain of his present life and the contact with so much suffering which he had little power to allay was becoming almost more than he could bear. It was obvious that he felt it a great relief to turn to the doctor from Claridge's for sympathy and comfort.

' Come and see the men,' he said.

They walked together to the church. The west door was open. The smell of sepsis and foul wounds met them as they entered the graveyard. Near the door some R.A.M.C. orderlies were tending a cooker, and on a bench a cheese stood among some long loaves and a few tins of Maconochie's ration. Packets of lint and cotton-wool were scattered on the ground, and some mugs and ration tins were piled in the porch. The floor of the church was covered with wounded men in ragged khaki. They lay upon straw close together.

Some of them were moaning quietly; others
muttered in their delirium. Some were dying as
the doctors stood near, and more than one had
entered into rest. The smell, the dirt and the
misery of it all was overwhelming. It was heart-
rending, too, to think of the women to whom
these men belonged. In the midst of such squalor
and wretchedness, an Army Sister, radiant in
scarlet and white, presented a strange contrast.

When ambulances could be spared, they came
down in the evening and carried as many wounded
as they could to a station—where the men waited
sometimes for days for a train. In this way they
were transported long distances, even to St.
Nazaire on their way to England. Such suffering !
Such loss of life ! And yet within sixty miles
lay Paris with thirty thousand empty beds, but
with no organised transport.

Dr. Garrett Anderson had two places in her
car, and she offered to take back with her two
wounded men who could sit up. Out of the
medley the orderlies produced two. They sat
them on a bench and washed their faces with
a piece of lint wrung out of the copper. They
put their caps on their heads, gave them a drink
of tea and intimated that they were ready. Dr.
Anderson looked at them, and it seemed to her

that one of them was too ill for the long drive in
an open car ; but when he saw that she was hesitating, the tears came into his eyes, and he caught
her arm, pleading :

' Do take me, lady. Don't leave me behind.'

So he had to be taken. She fortified them both
with a dose of morphia and some brandy diluted
with water from the copper ; then they were
helped into the car and driven away.

The memory of the men she had left in that
putrid atmosphere and under such comfortless
conditions was never to be forgotten.

No doubt some report of circumstances like
these reached the authorities in England. Towards the end of September, the War Office sent
over a representative to examine into existing
conditions, and to inspect and report on the
auxiliary hospitals, of which Claridge's Hôtel was
one. The ' Milord ' selected for this mission
made a handsome, martial figure as he strode
through the streets of Paris. He was resplendent
in khaki and brass hat, and a beautiful order hung
round his neck. Rumour said he was the Duke
of Connaught or Lord French or Sir Frederick
Treves or Mr. Bottomley ! But whoever he was,
his appearance commanded great respect. He

was saluted on all sides, and men stepped from
the pavement to let him take his noble way.

The first hospital which he visited was Claridge's.
He was an imposing figure as he entered the central
hall. His spurs rang on the pavement and his
steps re-echoed in its vastness. He fixed a sus-
picious blue eye on the senior medical officers who
went to meet him, and interrogated them sternly :

'Who is in charge of this place ?'

'What are you doing here ?'

'What have you got behind there ?' pointing
at the glass partition rendered opaque by white
paper.

'A French hospital ! How can it be a French
hospital ? You 're British.'

'All women ! No proper surgeons ?'

'Have you British soldiers here ? Any officers?'

'What are you doing with them ?'

'Where do they go when they leave you ?'

'Versailles ! Who told you to send them to
Versailles ?'

'Colonel Smith ! How do you know about
Colonel Smith ?'

Curt, sharp questions that met with curt, sharp
answers.

At this moment Madame Pérouse, who had been
notified of his visit, arrived. He greeted her with

D

the most delightful courtesy, and withdrawing with her to a little distance, asked if these women were really practical surgeons and if it were possible that the soldiers tolerated such an arrangement.

The poor old lady was rather flustered, but she declared that this was her 'meilleure installation' and that the organisation was 'parfaite.' He was only half-convinced by the assurances which she gave him, but his manner became more ordinary, and turning to Dr. Flora Murray and Dr. Garrett Anderson, he announced his intention of going through the wards. He was accompanied by a doctor, a civilian, whom he introduced as being 'unconverted to women doctors.' These pleasing preliminaries being concluded, he was conducted into the hospital.

It was the rest hour, when many of the patients were asleep, and an air of peace and comfort was over everything. Sisters moved softly whilst tending the more seriously ill, and those who were awake lay quietly reading and smoking. The handsome wards with their flowers and coloured blankets looked charming : for they were in perfect order, and there were no visitors so early in the day. The men when questioned spoke of their 'good home' with grateful appreciation.

The officers expressed their satisfaction in cordial
terms ; and as ' Milord ' went from ward to ward,
he became silent and thoughtful. He finished his
inspection without relaxing the severity of his
aspect and took a graceful farewell of Madame
Pérouse, leaving her much mystified as to the
reason of his visit and his apparent displeasure.

' Qu'est - ce   qu'il   avait ? '   she inquired.   ' Il
me semblait mécontent.'

Two days later the ' unconverted doctor ' called
again, bland and eager for conversation. He
explained that he and his companion had been
sent over by the War Office, and he talked of the
intentions of ' K ' with regard to the hospitals.
He said they wanted to know whether the Women's
Hospital Corps could increase its beds, and whether
it could move its hospital forward if needed.
The astonished organisers were given to understand that if any auxiliary hospitals were moved
forward, Claridge's would be the first to be invited
to move, and that the British Army would not
hesitate to make use of it, supposing that the
matter could be arranged with the French Red
Cross. The 'unconverted one' still seemed, however, to be tormented with uncertainty as to the
attitude of men when called upon to accept treatment from women doctors. In order to reassure

him, he was pressed to visit the officers' ward
by himself. He went, and, to the amusement of
all concerned, returned an agreeable and equable
convert.

Early in October 'Milord' was in Paris and
came to Claridge's again, bringing with him
Professor Alexis Thomson, of surgical fame and
of Edinburgh University. He greeted the staff
in the friendliest manner, and introducing the
Professor to them, he explained that he had
brought him because he believed that he would
be as much impressed as he himself had been.
He turned to the Professor and said :

'It's a curious thing, Thomson. They are all
lady doctors here. Have you ever come across
any ? '

'Yes, we begin with them at Edinburgh,' the
Professor replied. By which it was understood
that, as a junior member of the Infirmary staff,
it had been his duty to teach the women
students.

In the wards he was shown two trephined
patients who were doing well, and several compound fractures of thigh. He was interested to
see that Dr. Anderson was using Steinman's pins,
and discussed that method of treatment with her.

But what pleased him most, perhaps, was the reply of a Scotsman to his inquiries :

' Aw, A 'm fine. A tak' ma meat an' A get ma parritch in the morning. A 'm fine.'

On many future occasions ' Milord ' visited the hospitals of the Women's Hospital Corps, always as a welcome and honoured guest, distinguished by his courtesy and his kindness.

The medical staff of Claridge's had taken a good deal of trouble to find out the correct way of evacuating convalescent officers and men. There was no organisation in Paris at that time dealing with the transport to hospital or the discharge of British wounded, and it was only by chance that the Corps got into touch with the officer-in-charge of the Military Hospital, Versailles, and arranged to evacuate its patients through him. No proper instructions had been sent round to the auxiliary hospitals ; and in many cases patients had been discharged from hospital and allowed to proceed direct to England. The War Office termed this ' leakage,' and took ' the gravest view ' of such an irregular proceeding. Subsequently, an R.A.M.C. colonel was established in a neighbouring hotel to act as a central authority. The R.A.M.C. authorities always treated the Hôtel Claridge as though it were a British auxiliary ; whereas, in reality, it was affiliated to the French Military Hospital St. Martin. Troops of both nations used the hospital as long as it was open, and there was no difficulty in serving both masters. Inspection by highly placed officials of both Armies was constant ; and these visits were often a source of amusement to the medical staff.

Senior officers of the British Army seldom came to Paris without including the Women's Hospital in their round of inspection. Especial care was taken to receive these gentlemen with ceremony. The *Médecin-en-Chef* always took them round herself, and whenever possible the Chief Surgeon assisted too. Under such an escort they could not fail to see everything that it was desired they should see ; and often they saw it rose-coloured through the spectacles of the doctors themselves ! By the end of the tour they were full of admiration for ' a model hospital,' as they used to phrase it, and almost always asked :

' But why are you a French hospital ? You ought to be working with us.'

' The War Office would never look at women doctors,' was the reply.

' Oh, but that 's absurd ! ' they exclaimed.

'Look at the work you are doing. We must tell them about it.'

The hostesses passed the conversational ball from one to the other with skilful tact, intent on educating the officer in question in the work of medical women. They told him stories of the men and of their contentment, of surgical results, of the approval of high officials and of the work which other women doctors were doing during the war, until lifelong opinions began to give way.

'There are men who are extraordinarily prejudiced about women,' he would say. 'You may not have met them. But for myself I think it is a pity the R.A.M.C. should be so pig-headed.'

'Has Sloggett been to see you?' asked one Brass-hat, referring to the Director of Medical Services for the British Armies in France.

'No, he has not been here.'

'I wonder at that. Great man with the ladies, Sloggett.'

'I expect we are not his kind of ladies,' rejoined the doctor drily, to the great appreciation of her hearer.

'That 's a silly sort of badge you are wearing,' observed one lieutenant-colonel; for both the senior doctors were suffragists and wore the purple, white and green badge of their union. As their motto was 'Deeds not Words,' they never attempted propaganda even with their colleagues, and it was rare indeed for an officer to raise the subject with them.

'Oh! are you not in favour of Woman's Suffrage?' she asked.

'No, I am not,' he replied stoutly: 'Horrid women!'

'Somehow, I thought *you* would be.'

'What made you think I would be?' he asked, falling into the trap.

'Well, you are not a stupid man, and you have been about the world a lot. You seemed to me to be unusually open-minded.'

'Well, I won't go so far as to say I am against it, you know,' he conceded.

And then the argument started, amplified by facts and reasons which would have opened any mind, and which finally sent him off 'almost persuaded.'

An R.A.M.C. general in a responsible position called one day when the senior medical officers were out. He was received by another member of the medical staff, and assuming the semi-

jocular, semi-familiar attitude which professional
women dislike so much in their colleagues, permitted himself to say :

' I don't know anything about lady doctors.
Do you bite ? '

It was almost the only time that this sort of thing
was encountered. As a rule, there was no want
of courtesy ; and the doctors met with the kindest
consideration on all sides.

A more trying type of visitor was a celebrated
neurologist who, as he went round the wards,
looked over the patients as though they were
goods on a counter, and said in front of them :

' I want to see some good head cases. Have
you got anything shot through the brain ? Any
paralysis ? No fractures of skull ! Nothing good.
You don't seem to have much in. Deaf and dumb !
Hm—yes, that 's not bad. But I only want to
see head cases.'

To women who kept the human side very much
to the front this attitude was unsympathetic.
They much preferred the stout old chief from the
Hôpital St. Martin, who hated to see the French
soldiers without their *képis* on, even when in bed,
and who puffed himself out and frowned and
said that the hospital was ' curieux,' but sent
cases in all the same.

Each day seemed to bring fresh visitors. Amongst them were the American Ambassador and his predecessor, French *députés*, English Members of Parliament, Miss Jane Harrison, Mrs. Pankhurst, Lord Robert Cecil, Lord Lytton, French ladies and gentlemen, English and American people resident in or passing through Paris and representatives of the Press of all the allied nations.

The minds of the French journalists were severely exercised on the subject of operations; for they could not believe that women were equal to such work. It was one thing to ' soigner les blessés ' and another to operate. It was conceivable that women might succeed as nurses; but as surgeons ! never ! These gentlemen would go admiringly over the hospital, listening to what the doctors told them and talking to the French patients, and then, before leaving, they would beg for permission to ask one more question. It was always the same question :

' Who is it really who operates ? '

One editor, to whom the surgeons were indicated in person, contemplated with serious attention Dr. Cuthbert, who was young and pleasing, and then said to her :

' Et vous, mademoiselle, vouz coupez aussi ? '

'Oui, je coupe,' she replied slowly; for her facility with the knife was greater than with the French tongue.

'Incroyable!' he gasped.

For the most part, 'épatant' was the word they used, and the older journalists would listen silently and shake their heads incredulously.

The editor and assistant editor of *Le Matin* were so difficult to convince, that the *Médecin-en-Chef* offered to let them see the interior of the operating theatre, where work was going on. The assistant editor eagerly accepted the offer, and gazed spellbound through the screen which divided the anæsthetist's room from the theatre. He became so absorbed that it was difficult to get him to come away before the surgeon discovered and resented his presence. Once outside, he flung his arms round his chief and in an ecstasy of delight cried:

'Je l'ai vue—je l'ai vue—le couteau à la main!'

The reporters from the English papers wrote charming articles and paragraphs about the hospital, which were fruitful in rousing interest at home, and which brought subscriptions and many parcels to further the work.

CHAPTER VI

THE HOSPITAL AND ITS VISITORS

A LARGE sign was stretched across the portico of the Hôtel :

HÔPITAL ANGLO-BELGE,
173 AUXILIAIRE.

On Sunday afternoon, when all the world walked in the Champs Élysées, it attracted a great deal of notice. And M. Aubry, smoking his cigarette on the doorstep, was gratified by many inquiries about ' les blessés ' and the hospital.

With characteristic affability he bowed and made every one welcome, and sent a stream of unknown and curious people to see the wards. The visitors made him so many compliments upon his ' installation si parfaite ' that the following Sunday found him again on the doorstep. Before long he was surrounded by a large and friendly crowd ; for all who had seen the hospital the previous week had returned, bringing with them their families and friends to enjoy the ' épatant ' spectacle ! Even M. Aubry perceived

that it was impracticable to admit a seething
mass of two hundred or more people ; and the
staff promptly came to his support and closed
the grille in the face of a protesting, gesticulating
throng. After this incident, M. Aubry was persuaded to smoke elsewhere on Sundays.

The wards were visited regularly by many kind
friends, who took infinite trouble to get to know
the men personally and entertained them with
talk or reading. The Rev. Mr. Blunt, of the
British Embassy Church, came often, and his
curate, Mr. W. Bennett, was a daily visitor.
The latter visited the sick and talked football
round the brazzeros whilst he roasted chestnuts
and made toast. On Sundays he held a service,
with the help of the Baroness Geysa de Braunecker
and Mrs. Henley, who made music for the hospital
every evening. Their sing-songs in the big central
hall were delightful : English songs, Scotch songs,
French songs, one after the other. ' Tipperary '
was the favourite then, but ' Thora ' had a great
vogue, and a heavy bass would thrill the company
with :

' Speak ! speak ! speak to me, Thora ! '
Most popular, too, was ' The Bonnie Banks of Loch
Lomond.' And the ' Marseillaise ' united every-
body in one great roar.

A natural comedian among the patients, called Ginger by his comrades on account of the colour of his hair, mounted the platform readily to give his song : ' With my little wiggle waggle in my hand.' He received so many encores that he felt encouraged to make a speech. He began by saying how much he enjoyed the appreciation of the audience because he knew how well he deserved it ; and then he wandered off into praise of his feats with the Army, ending up with kindly comments on the comfort of the hospital.

From the neighbouring church of S. Philippe du Roule came l'Abbé Charles Ablin to care for the Roman Catholics. M. l'Abbé was as tenderhearted and sympathetic as St. Francis himself. His spiritual face radiated gentleness and piety. His heart ached for the wounded and the dying. To go round a screen with him and see him raise his hands and murmur, ' Ah ! nos braves, nos braves ! ' called up a vision of suffering, bleeding France. In every delirious or dying infantryman he saw his country, and he poured out his love and pity on each one. He lamented that he could not speak to the English, but he visited them all the same : ' At least I can bless them,' he said.

And day by day he passed among them, raising his hand and murmuring gentle words : so that they learned to love him, and missed him if he did not come. He had his own anxieties too ; for a niece who lived with him had gone to a Belgian convent for a holiday in August, and he had had no news of her since the war broke out. In January he heard that she had reached England, and in a tremor of joy and relief he set out for London to bring her home.

Mr. Chester Fentress, the well-known tenor, was at that time living in Paris. When the work on which he was engaged at the American Embassy came to an end, he found that the American hospital had more workers than it needed, and fortunately he was able to attach himself to ' Claridge's.' He came every day, ready to do anything, until he was regarded as an orderly of the Corps, and helping in the wards he suffered some things at the hands of the Sisters and patients.

' There is a lamp there,' one Sister was heard to say to him. ' I cannot get it to burn. Would you have the sense now to put it right ? '

Nor was his genius always recognised ! An irritable patient, hearing him sing as he performed some menial task, exclaimed :

' God help him, if he had to earn his living by his voice ! '

Mr. Fentress's knowledge of Paris and of the

shops was of great use. He was an expert shopper and guide, and very kind about undertaking commissions. Later in the autumn he brought his friend, Mr. Hubert Henry Davies, the playwright, to the hospital, and made him so interested that when work pressed and helpers were few he also would don a white coat and enter the wards. It appealed to his sense of fun to fetch and carry for the Sisters, and the men were a constant interest and pleasure to him. He was dearly loved by everybody for his sensitive nature, his refinement, his humour and the way in which he threw himself into the hospital life.

Amongst the nurses was one elderly lady who had once nursed for Mrs. Garrett Anderson and who never failed to impress the fact on any doctor who ventured to comment on disorder or want of management in her ward. If reminded that the men should breakfast at 8 A.M. and not 9 A.M., she would reply :

' Well, I have nursed for Mrs. Garrett Anderson, and she always said it was a mistake for patients to breakfast early.'

If it were pointed out that dinner was over in other wards and had not yet begun in hers, the answer was :

' When I nursed for Mrs. Garrett Anderson, she

always said that patients should not be pressed to eat till they were hungry.'

If asked to put an extra jacket on the man whose bed was near the passage way, the doctor was informed :

'Mrs. Garrett Anderson did not approve of muffling up patients, and I nursed for her long enough to know.'

Or she would remark crushingly :

'Well, doctors are not what they were when I nursed for Mrs. Garrett Anderson.'

The medical staff bore itself humbly, for it was already conscious of its inferiority to the great Pioneer ; and try as they might, they never succeeded in learning when and where the nurse had had this great experience. Her quaint habits of mind and plainness of speech made her a joy to Mr. Davies. Meeting him one day on the Boulevards, she attacked him for not having emptied her dressing-bin that morning, and drew such a pathetic picture of her plight in consequence of his negligence that she moved herself to tears. Both he and Mr. Fentress were horrified to find themselves and the weeping nurse objects of public interest. They hastily pushed her into the nearest shop, hoping to propitiate her with coffee. But the shop turned out to be a bookshop, and she

E

never read books. It took some time before a
suitable offering could be found and friendly
relations be re-established.

Nearly every afternoon saw Lady Robert Cecil
in the wards. She was always a most welcome
visitor. No one knew better than she did how
to make the time pass pleasantly. Mrs. Kemp
came too, with generous supplies of English
bread, which the men regarded as a great treat
after the French loaves. And at Christmas time
Mrs. Pankhurst was in Paris, and her first visit
made an equal sensation among French and British.
They would gather round her while she talked to
them of their homes and the education of their
children, or encouraged them to consider how
the heavy daily toil of their wives might be
lightened.

' I would rather have seen that lady than that
Queen who came the other day,' said one, referring to the visit of Queen Amelie of Portugal.
And the roughest diamond, a bricklayer, not unaccustomed to beer drinking, delivered himself:

' I do declare to you, lady, that this war has
shown me that the " spear " of woman is something different to what I thought it had been.'

But very often there were more visitors than
was desirable ; men suffered from too much

attention and grew weary of the repeated inquiries as to wounds and progress. The sick would gladly accept the suggestion to have screens put round them, and even then they were not always safe from intrusion. A lady in 'a shepherd's plaid frock' upset a Cameron Highlander by commenting on his lemonade and grapes and calling him 'one of the pampered ones.'

'I would have ye know, mem,' he retorted, 'I'm a Brrritish soldier man and not a toy dog. What should I want to be pampered for more nor other men—and me a Cameron ? '

And to his nurse afterwards he confided :

'She fair maks me seeck.'

Two days later the same tactless lady again gave him cause for complaint.

'She offered me a cake an' I took it, for she was vera polite. An' then she starts her sauce. "There's naething the matter wi' ye," she says. An' I says, "Ye're right, there's naething wrang wi' me an' so I'm no' needing ony mair visitors." An' I never touched her cake ; I'll never touch her cake again—wi' her shepherd's tartan frock an' a',' he growled wrathfully.

At a later stage the Cameron was met in a corridor, with his uninjured arm fondling a Belgian girl. The doctor who met him remarked upon his affectionate manner.

'Och, Doctor, she's got the toothache an' I canna speak French.' And in complete understanding they wandered undisturbed down the corridor.

It was difficult to make kindly - intentioned people understand that the wards must close at certain hours or that the men were really ill and must have quiet. Concert parties and people with views on recitation would arrive unexpectedly at a late hour, and fail to see any reason why performances could not be given during supper or with the sleeping draughts. A lady brought a French poet to recite his works to a ward which held principally Englishmen, at the time when general washing and blanket bathing was in full swing. The sight alone of the poet caused catastrophes among the basins; for his appearance was as advanced as his verse, and his long hair and bow tie and very full-skirted coat were more than startling to British eyes.

Other hospital units, waiting in Paris for a location, called to see round Claridge's, and amongst such visitors were the Duchess of Westminster, Lady Sarah Wilson and Lady Dudley. The surgeons belonging to these units were restive at being kept waiting so long and inclined to be envious of the Women's Hospital Corps, which had been running for some weeks; but their hospitals had a large personnel, for which quarters were not so easy to find as they had been for the women's smaller unit.

In December a cordial welcome was extended to Dr. Elsie Inglis and Dr. Frances Ivens, who, with a Scottish Women's Hospital, were on their way to L'Abbaye Royaumont, to open the hospital which became so famous. At an earlier date Dr. Elsie Inglis had written to Dr. Garrett Anderson to ask if there were a vacancy for a surgeon in the Women's Hospital Corps; but the Unit had its full complement of surgeons; and her suggestion to join it was regretfully declined. In view of what she afterwards initiated and accomplished, this was not the matter of regret which it seemed at the time. It was splendid to have another women's hospital established under the French Red Cross, and to hear also of the other Scottish units which were going farther afield.

The presence of their English colleagues was stimulating to the French medical women, and they did not fail to contrast their own position unfavourably with that accorded to their foreign sisters. Whereas English women were established in control of hospitals under the French Red Cross, the French women were serving in military hospitals as dressers, or as night orderly officers. They had no responsible work, and no professional position. One afternoon, Madame Paul Boyer brought a number of them to ' Claridge's,' when a free discussion took place over the coffee cups.

Although the Paris University had opened its degree to women many years before the Universities of the United Kingdom, the number of women on the register fell far below the number in England. Educational facilities were equal in Paris for men and women, but after qualification the resident posts and staff appointments were still given to men, and women could only secure very subordinate work. They were not combined in any society, as the British women are. They had no association or council to promote their interests, and they had no hospitals of their own, staffed and supported by women, through which they might obtain responsible surgical work and experience.

When war broke out, their Government scorned their offer of service, and it was only as the result of the shortage of doctors that a few had obtained any footing at all in military hospitals.   Dr. N.-K., a Russian lady of great ability and many years' experience, was working as a dresser under a lieutenant of twenty-two years in the officers' section at 'St. Louis.'   Her work seemed to be largely that which a nurse would do in England. She took temperatures, dressed wounds, kept notes, directed the male orderlies, but was denied all responsibility in professional matters.   Mme. Boyer was permitted to sleep in the 'Val de Grace' and attend to night calls.   She lamented the absence of women, whether as nurses or doctors, in the French hospitals, and described in graphic terms the confusion and discomfort to be found there.   Another, who spoke Polish, had been told that she might join a hospital on the eastern frontier if she were disguised as an *infirmière*, but that she must promise not to disclose to the *Médecin-en-Chef* that she was a doctor.

Most of these women doctors were married and very much domesticated, but they complained unanimously of having no opportunities, and were even a little bitter about the unfairness of their position.   Dr. Garrett Anderson and Dr. Flora Murray pointed out that women must make their own opportunities, and told them of the societies, schools and hospitals for women in England. At last, stirred to emulate, they declared that they also must 'faire un mouvement.' Then one said that her husband did not like her to concern herself with 'mouvements,' and another that, if a 'mouvement' meant attending meetings at night, she could not come, because her husband could not bear to be left alone. And the enthusiasm began to dwindle. Pressed to consider the possibility of a hospital staffed by women, they admitted that it would be an advantage, and that such a scheme might be feasible, till Mme. Boyer said that they had had no chance of surgical experience and asked dramatically what they should do 'if the first patient came with an *énorme fibrome*.'

But there were at least two silent onlookers, young women, one of whom had not yet finished her medical course but knew English, had been in England and had some knowledge of the women's movement there. She and her comrade were not married, and they obviously had personal ambition. They had been touched by the modern spirit. Through them and through their contemporaries progress might come. They sat listening to their seniors with decorum and in silence. But their eyes were critical and in

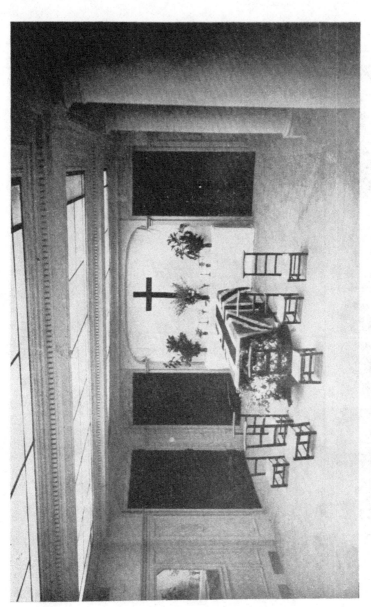

THE MORTUARY IN THE HÔTEL CLARIDGE

(Page 74)

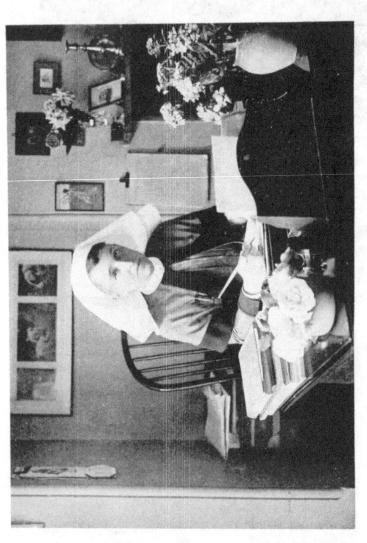

THE MATRON OF THE MILITARY HOSPITAL, ENDELL STREET. (Page 75)
MISS G. R. HALE, R.R.C.

(Photo, Reginald Haines)

their hearts they judged them and found them wanting.

The English doctors realised that the new element was present, and that the advance had sounded for professional women in France.

CHAPTER VII

LES DÉFENSEURS DE NOTRE PATRIE

THE rate of mortality was lamentably high, for the men coming into the hospital were not only badly wounded, but also in bad condition ; and tetanus and gas gangrene, shock and sepsis claimed their victims. The recovery of the French soldiers was hindered by the painful impression made on them by the invasion of their country. In delirium or under the anæsthetic they raved of their *patrie,* of her beauty and of their love for her ; and horror and fear of the German dominated their minds. The men who owned and loved the soil spoke on their deathbeds always and only of France. They were tormented with anxiety for her safety and welfare ; and the mental agony which they endured lessened their vitality and power of resistance.

The mortuary was arranged in the hall which had been designed for a grill-room. It had a separate entrance from the street, and was lit by a beautiful 'plafond lumière.' Departed heroes,

surrounded by flowers, lay before the temporary
altar : the laurel wreath was not wanting ; nor
was reverent care from their countrywomen
lacking.

Funerals were arranged to leave the hospital at
8 A.M. For some of them the chaplain came to the
hospital to read the first part of the Service in
the Chapel ; for others this was read in the Church
of S. Philippe du Roule. In the sunshine of the
autumn mornings an attentive, sympathetic little
crowd used to gather round the entrance of the
Hôtel. The coffin would be placed on an open
hearse, and covered by the national flag of the
soldier who lay there. A picket of soldiers and a
detachment of police accompanied the hearse,
and the undertaker in evening dress, with cocked
hat and blue and red scarf of office, led the way.
The police laid palms on the coffin, tied with a
broad ribbon, on which was inscribed : ' Pour les
Défenseurs de notre Patrie ' ; and another wreath
was sent by the military authorities. It was made
of bead flowers with a plate, on which was written :
' Souvenir français ' for the British soldiers, and
' À notre Brave qui est mort pour la patrie ' for
the French. Members of the staff accompanied
the hearse. Sometimes M. Aubry went too, or
the hairdresser from across the way, for he learnt

to know the men by coming regularly and grat-
uitously to shave them. Constantly a little old
lady attended, English by birth and French by
habit. She was aged and poor; and the only
war service within her power was that of following
British soldiers to the grave. No one knew how
she heard that a death had occurred; but she
constantly arrived with a rose blessed by the
Pope to lay in the coffin, and a request to be told
the hour next morning. The orderlies used to
say that she looked disappointed if they told her
that men who were seriously ill were better. Be
that as it may, she was faithful in the service she
had laid down for herself; and her pathetic little
figure, in straw bonnet and much worn sealskin
jacket, was seldom absent when the sad procession
started from the Hôtel.

In the autumn of 1914 eight o'clock was Paris's
most beautiful hour: the newly watered Champs
Elysées shone blue with the reflection of the sky,
and the leaves on the lime trees shone gold in the
sunlight. As the hearse made its way to the
church, women ran to lay flowers on the coffin,
men stood in silent salute, and the pious crossed
themselves and said a prayer.

On the steps of the church the beadle stood
waiting, a wonderful presence, six foot high and

corpulent, impressive in his laced coat and three-cornered hat, and bearing a staff of ebony topped by a large silver knob. He marched up the church in front of the procession, rattling his staff on the stones at every third step, and continued during the service to act as director and usher. The services were held in the Lady Chapel, and at intervals his staff would rattle on the aisle, and with a bow to either side he would give directions ' s'asseoir, messieurs et mesdames.'

After the service the hospital staff waited in the side aisle whilst the coffin was carried out, and at these times kindly old people came to ask about the dead soldier. Was he English or French ? wounded or sick ? Had he a wife and children ? How many *blessés* lay in the hospital ?

And benedictions, gratitude and five - franc pieces were bestowed upon ' les dames anglaises.'

In the cemetery of St. Pantin, outside Paris, the rows of graves and wooden crosses increased in number, and French and British side by side lay at rest.

CHAPTER VIII

THE UNIT EXPANDS

THE number of patients coming into a war hospital must inevitably fluctuate, and ' Claridge's ' had its easy as well as its heavy periods. During September and the first half of October the wards were occupied principally by British wounded ; but as the weeks went on, the War Office completed its arrangements, and hospital trains were sent down to transport the men to England, and fewer came into Paris. Meanwhile, affiliation with a French military hospital had taken place, and a greater number of French sick and wounded were sent in, as well as some Belgians. November brought a lull, and the wards became comparatively empty. An R.A.M.C. general called and asked that a hundred and fifty beds might be made ready, as it was intended to send large numbers of light cases to Paris, but the expected trains did not arrive till December, when once more every available bed was filled by the British.

Investigation revealed that the reduction of French admissions was caused by difficulties which had arisen between the Red Cross offices in the rue de Thann and the Governor of Paris. The Red Cross *directeur*, M. le Dr. M——, was of a choleric disposition; and when he insulted the military authorities, they retaliated by cutting all the rue de Thann hospitals off the station list. Hospitals which were not on this list did not receive any wounded, even though they sent their ambulances with a *permis* signed by M. le Dr. M——. New regulations, too, were constantly made; so that the papers which had been in order on Monday might be obsolete on Wednesday. After one of these inimical passages it was decreed that ambulances must carry a *permission* from the *Service de Santé* in addition to the Red Cross mandate. The rue de Thann was not successful in obtaining the necessary document from headquarters, and consequently M. Falcouz suggested that Dr. Flora Murray should go in person to see the Governor and ask for an authority from him.

It transpired that appointments were not made with M. le Général F——. The usual procedure was to be on the steps of his *cabinet* at eight o'clock in the morning. He held a *Réunion* at seven o'clock every morning; and those who wished for interviews waited to catch him when the *Réunion* dispersed.

M. le Général was very handsome : six foot in
height, he was broad in proportion and his red
and blue uniform was highly becoming. As he
stood on the steps shaking hands with his colleagues, he was a debonair and pleasant figure.
There was power in his face and a sense of humour,
but there was cunning too. His extreme courtesy
did not completely disguise his insincerity. He
was frankly curious about the women doctors, but
behind his polite interest was scepticism. Dr.
Murray presented a letter of introduction from a
British official, and requested M. le Général to
furnish her with the necessary authority for the
stations and an order for coal and coke. Experience had shown that he was always ready to
promise everything that he was asked, but that
his promises were seldom fulfilled. With great
affability he said that he would send the author-
isation and that he would refer the question of
coal to ' l'intendance militaire.' It was to meet
this contingency that Orderly Hodgson had accompanied the doctor. She said she would wait
and take both papers with her.

' It will take an hour to prepare,' said the
secretary.

' I will wait an hour,' she said amiably.

' It may perhaps be two hours,' he warned her.

'I will wait two hours,' she said, still more amiably.

'Or perhaps till *midi*,' he insisted.

'It is well. I will wait till *midi*,' she rejoined.

He shrugged his shoulders and invited her to follow him to his office. Before letting Dr. Murray go, M. le Général entered into his reasons for requiring thirty thousand beds in Paris, and ended with :

'Je tiens absolument à retenir votre installation.'

Probably he did not care at all, but he feared that if he let the hospital leave Paris the British would absorb it. The interview was useful. The necessary document was granted ; and for a time obstruction ceased.

The French soldiers who were admitted to the hospital were in a much worse condition than the British. To begin with, they were of a more intellectual and imaginative temperament, and they suffered in mind as well as in body. They had borne great hardships, for their clothing and equipment, and especially their commissariat, fell far below the British standard.

One of those admitted was Pte. Darcy of the *Légion étrangère.* He was one of several hundred young Englishmen resident in Paris who, on the

F

outbreak of war, had precipitately joined the French Army. When wounded, he insisted on being put out of the train near Paris, that he might go to an English hospital. As he recovered, he told how he had joined in a hurry because he feared that he would miss all the fighting if he went home and went through his training. He described his experiences with the French Army: the severe training of recruits, the inadequate accommodation, the lack of bedding, clothing, food, and the indifferent medical attention. In the trenches his regiment remained unrelieved for long periods, and for weeks his food was bread and a sardine. Both he and his brother had married French women and lived in Paris. His brother had been shell-shocked and was deaf and dumb, and being unable to protest, had been re-moved to a French hospital in the provinces. With a good deal of trouble his transfer to Clar-idge's was effected ; and the two brothers had beds side by side and were very happy in their reunion.

Other men in the ward became much interested in the cure of ' Darcy's brother,' as every one called him, and combined to stand behind him and yell all together, to try and make him hear. The din was terrible, but it gave the whole ward

great pleasure ; and when at last, one evening,
Darcy's brother heard and turned round and
smiled at them, they cheered vociferously. Soon
after this he recovered his speech also ; and, in
his delight, it seemed to the staff as though from
that moment he never ceased talking.

They came from all over France, these men—
from north and south, from the Pyrénées and the
Vosges : Zouaves, Moroccans, Bretons, Alsatians
—with their various types and uniforms, and,
what was more embarrassing, with their various
patois. The nurses learnt their tastes in food and
in wine ; they studied the difference in their
temperaments ; prepared tisanes and special
dishes, and made them all happy and at home.
A simple Poilu could not sleep at night for wonder
and delight at being in a marble hall. His melan-
choly neighbour answered every inquiry about
his arm with ' Ça pique ; ça pique toujours.'
Sergeant Jacquot had innumerable smart lady
friends. And ' le Caporal ' had quaint old parents
from the Midi, who travelled all night to come and
see him and bring him a cheese and raisin wine.

The French soldier associated with the British
very readily, joining in his games and songs as
though the difference of language was no impedi-
ment to understanding. He was the most grateful

and appreciative of patients—glad to be nursed,
massaged and well treated. Only, now and then,
he would say :

' Our hospitals are not like that.'

This was the only criticism of his country's
institutions that ever escaped him ; for his
patience under hardship was wonderful. His
thick red trousers were always too large for him ;
his heavy long blue coat was most cumbersome,
and his boots left much to be desired. His under-
clothing was of cotton ; and he might or might
not have socks with which to face the damp and
cold in the trenches. But he was a valiant and
an intrepid fighter, and his intense patriotism
made him the most uncomplaining and enduring
of men.

Some of those who found refuge at Claridge's
had been shelled out of three hospitals and had
lain on straw in a cellar for six weeks. Others had
homes in the occupied area and did not know
what had become of their wives and families.
Most of them had closed their shops and left their
business, and their future was uncertain. But,
one and all, they were certain of victory, and confidently referred to the time when the German
should be beaten.

The hardships of the winter and the wet climate

told very heavily upon the Algerians, who reached
hospital in a miserable condition. They were
the victims of severe frostbite, and in one case,
at any rate, both feet had to be amputated. This
man remained in the hospital for a considerable
time. Mrs. Kemp, who visited his ward, was very
kind in bringing fruit to him and his compatriots,
for they loved to consume large quantities of it.
One day she asked him what he would like for a
present, and he said that his desire was to possess
a valise. He received it, when she brought it,
with wide smiles. It was covered with grey
cloth, and had shiny black leather straps and
handles and was considered very attractive. At
the earliest opportunity he summoned his doctor
to his bedside, and showing her the valise, asked
for his feet. Alas ! they had not been preserved,
and he was bitterly disappointed.

When reports reached Paris of the heavy fighting in the north and of the great rush of wounded
to Boulogne, the English hospitals in that city
made up a party of surgeons and nurses and sent
them to give any additional aid which might be
required. Three doctors from ' Claridge's ' were
of the party. When they reached Boulogne
they found the hospitals and stations seriously

overcrowded, and approximately three thousand casualties were coming in daily. The authorities, however, refused all outside help. They said that they had ample staff and needed no volunteers; and it was even supposed that orders were given to refuse civilians access to the hospitals.

The women doctors made friends with the matron of one of the hospitals, who told them that she had orders not to take any doctors round; but as they were women and in uniform, they would probably pass as nurses, and therefore she would show them some of the wards. They found the accommodation had been stretched to the uttermost. Instead of four hundred patients there were eight hundred. Rows of stretchers filled the corridors, and the orderlies were stepping over the men in their efforts to pass water or food among them. The dressings could not be overtaken. The men were unwashed, and in many cases their dressings had not been changed for days, owing to want of staff. They lay in Boulogne for two or three days, and were then transferred to England. Everywhere there was overcrowding, and it was evident that more hospitals were needed.

The next day the officer in charge of one of the hospitals, finding himself hopelessly short-handed, asked for the temporary assistance of two women surgeons. Dr. Rosalie Jobson and Dr. Marjorie Blandy were accordingly lent to him by the Corps. They became attached to his staff and remained serving under the R.A.M.C. in this post for six months. During this time the Corps maintained them, the Army accepting their services gratis.

Acting on instructions from Paris, Dr. Gazdar called at the headquarters of the Army Medical Service, and found that the Women's Hospital Corps was well known. She stated that the Corps proposed to establish another hospital in Boulogne, and asked whether it would be welcome to the authorities.

In reply, she was told :

' If you had a place here, we should certainly use you. We know all about your work in Paris.'

She then returned to Paris, where preparations were already being made for the second hospital. The French Red Cross was willing that the Unit should divide and extend its sphere of work, so long as it bore the expense itself. And M. Falcouz offered them all assistance in obtaining transport for the heavy luggage and permission to move the ambulances, which Mlle Block and Miss Grey were anxious should go with them.

On the 1st of November Dr. Garrett Anderson

and Dr. Flora Murray left for Boulogne, to find a
house for the new hospital and get it ready for
occupation.

The company in the very crowded railway
carriage in which they travelled included a lady
and gentleman who had fled from Lille and who
were going to Calais. Madame had what she
called ' un petit panier ' on her knee, and very
politely hoped it would not inconvenience her
fellow-passengers. The *panier* measured twenty-
eight by thirty-six inches and contained two dainty
little dogs. These howled whenever Madame left
the compartment, and she left it frequently,
for she was stout and the carriage was airless.
When they howled, Monsieur beat on the lid of the
panier and called them *bêtes* and *infâmes*.

In one corner a French woman who had been
nursing in a hospital for the wounded recounted
her experiences. She related how a German had
lain in the hospital, with both hands helpless ;
and how the nurses had always attended to him
last ; how she herself, when she did anything for
him, always said :

' I do not do this for my own pleasure, but
because God has so commanded me.'

And the carriage nodded its head in approval.
Further, she described how, being set to feed him

with rice and milk, she made this remark with each mouthful ; till, goaded beyond bearing, the man spat the food out in her face. And the carriage exclaimed with horror at the brute. Then all the nurses gathered round to tell him what they thought of him, and unanimously declared they would refuse ever to feed him again. The *infirmière majeure*, being informed, said that she would feed him, and with the spoon and basin she approached the bed. The poor man, however, let himself go and ejected the rice and milk thus bestowed upon him in the direction of the lady herself. The carriage lifted its hands in horror, and agreed, as the raconteur continued, that after that there was nothing more to be done, and the *Médecin-en-Chef* had to remove the wounded German.

With such tales the long journey was beguiled.

CHAPTER IX

THE HOSPITAL AT WIMEREUX UNDER THE R.A.M.C.
IS OPENED

In Boulogne itself every place which was suitable
for hospital purposes was already occupied, but
there was a large house at Wimereux which was
to let. The little town was full of jerry-built
hotels and chalets, erected by the *maire* and rented
in times of peace to the summer visitors, who were
a source of revenue both to him and to the town.
The large hotels were all let to the Army, but the
Château Mauricien was vacant ; and although it
was Sunday, the agent was prepared to do business.

The château had originally been built by an
Englishman, and it was provided with an English
cooking range and hot-water system as well as
with central heating. Its chief attractions were
its position in the eye of the sun, with a large
garden all round it, and the purity and freshness
of the air. Attached to it was a three-storied
dépendance, which promised quarters for the staff.
In addition the stable, coach-house, garage and

greenhouses could all be made use of. It is true
that the roof was inclined to leak and that the
drainage system was obsolete and broke down
hopelessly ; but the place was full of sunshine
and sweetness, and made a passable hospital
both then and later.

The agent, M. Jean Bataille, who acted for the
maire, had the appearance and manners of a bluff
sea-captain. His appearance suggested that his
blue serge clothing covered an honest heart, that
his mind was as guileless as a child's, and that
philanthropy was his hobby. He had a fixed idea
that to be English was to be wealthy ; and experience had shown him that in matters of business
the English were as babes in the hands of the
maire and himself. Between them they monopo-
lised most of the trades and all the public offices of
the town ; nothing could be obtained and very
little could be done without applying to the
maire. Builders, chimney-sweeps, plumbers, gas-
fitters—all seemed to be his employees. No one
else had houses or hotels to let. The milk came
from his farm ; the coal through his agency. He
controlled *l'apparat* by which the congestion of
drains was relieved ; and by virtue of his office
he issued requisition orders and *autorités* at his
own discretion and his own price.

The greater part of the morning was spent in argument, on the sunny terrace of the château, before the bargain was struck. The terms of the *maire* were high, and he haggled and held out ; but finally, having been assured that the Légion d'honneur was likely to be his, and that his association with the British Army might bring further honours, he melted, and agreed to put the house in order and let it to the Women's Hospital Corps for six weeks, or longer if they wanted it. The party adjourned to the *maire's* office—a black little den behind his house—so that the agreement might be drawn up. There was only standing room in the office, and a board laid on the top of the stove acted as a writing table ! M. le Maire and M. Bataille were unable to write more than their own names, and the agreement had to be composed and written by the doctors themselves. With much concentration and deep breathing the gentlemen affixed their signatures. The document being completed, they beamed on the ladies, and promised to have workmen and cleaners in the house by sunrise next day.

By ten o'clock in the morning the sweep, the plumber and the gas-fitter had not arrived ; the women who were to do the cleaning were still absent, and the *maire* himself was invisible. The

town had to be turned upside down to discover
them all ; and when once they were set to work,
it was necessary to stand by and keep a watchful
eye upon them, lest they should disappear and
get lost again.

The château needed furniture. And here the
maire was supreme ; for he had stores of furniture
stacked in the ' Salle Jeanne d'Arc,' which he
had removed from the Grand Hotel when he let
it to the R.A.M.C. for a hospital. He was charmed
that it should be requisitioned, and the agent
sent two ramshackle old carts and a couple of
men to convey mattresses and tables and chairs
from the *salle* to the new hospital. Through him
also a *batterie de cuisine* was unearthed from the
underground cellars of the Grand Hotel ; and
from cupboards in the typhoid wards cutlery and
knives and forks were forthcoming. With the
supplies and stores from Paris, and others which
Dr. Woodcock sent over, the château assumed a
fairly habitable and comfortable appearance.
There was no furniture available for the staff ;
for the *maire* lent on hire at exorbitant rates ;
and therefore they contented themselves with
mattresses on the floor of the *dépendance* for many
weeks, until the British Red Cross came to their
relief with bedsteads.

Dr. Cuthbert arrived from Paris with a detachment of nurses and orderlies, who soon brought order into the house. And, to every one's joy, Miss Fenn and Miss Goodwin, professional cook and parlour-maid, came over from London to run the establishment. After the arrangements at Claridge's, English cooking and ample army rations almost constituted luxury.

For the *service* some Belgian girls were engaged, and a French-English vocabulary was pinned on the kitchen wall, by means of which Miss Fenn and Miss Goodwin were able to direct the work. After a few days, a complete understanding took place between them; and cheerful conversation was not wanting.

For heavier work, one 'Joseph' was added to the establishment. He was a young Belgian of military age, who had no taste for military service! He was a refugee with his wife and child. He roused the sympathies of the staff by relating the graphic story of the death of his brother, whom he said he had seen cut into small pieces by German soldiers 'before his very eyes.'

'My only brother,' he would say, and burst into tears.

Much kindness was shown to his wife and little girl; and Joseph's own shortcomings and disappearances were leniently treated. A few weeks later he told the quartermaster with much indignation that his brother had written him a begging letter.

'But,' said the quartermaster, 'I thought you had only one brother ? '

'It is true, mam'selle, and now he wishes to beg of me.'

'But you said that you saw the Germans cut him to pieces,' remonstrated the quartermaster.

'It is true, mam'selle. Nevertheless, he has written asking me for money,' replied Joseph, too much absorbed in his anger against his brother to notice his own want of veracity.

The town was full of Belgians, for whom relief was organised by M. Larensard, the proprietor of the stationer's shop and library. He had a soup-kitchen in the coach-house of the château, and begged that he might not be displaced. He came daily to supervise the *soupe,* looking like an El Greco grandee, with his long ivory face, his pointed beard and erect white hair. He wore black clothes, a white clerical - looking tie and fluffy yellow socks, and on his arm a white brassard indicated his merciful calling. He had a Christian creed and lived up to it.

Dr. Flora Murray had brought letters of introduction with her from Paris, and as the preparations for the hospital were nearing completion, accompanied by Dr. Garrett Anderson, she called at the headquarters of the Army Medical Service in Boulogne and presented the letters. In a bare little hotel bedroom with a hideous French wallpaper on the walls, they found two colonels and a soldiers' table. The senior officer glanced at the correspondence and said :

' We know all about the Women's Hospital Corps here. Saw you in Paris. You are very welcome here. Have you got a place ? How many beds can you give us ? '

He seemed satisfied when the doctors answered that their ' place ' with a hundred beds would be ready next day. In answer to their inquiry whether he would make use of it, he said :

' Yes, to the fullest extent. I am Commandant here. You will be working directly under me. Will you take surgery ? We need another operating station.'

Their hearts leapt within them ; for all the time it had been their ambition to see women doctors working as army surgeons under the British War Office.

The conversation then took the form of instructions about registers, returns, reports and nominal rolls. The question of maintenance was discussed ; and it was proposed to provide the hospital with rations and coal, as well as petrol for its ambulances.

' Have you a quartermaster ? ' he asked.

' Yes, we have one,' Dr. Garrett Anderson replied, mentally appointing Orderly Campbell to this post as she spoke.

It was arranged that the Château Mauricien should be attached to the Military Hospital in the Grand Hotel, and that the newly appointed quartermaster should understudy the quartermaster of that hospital. An official document was issued for her use :

To O. i/c. Supplies.

The Women's Hospital Corps have established a hospital at the Château Mauricien at Wimereux, and is recognised by the War Office.

(Signed) D. D. S.——, Lt.-Col.,
for A. D. M. S.

5th November 1914.

Armed with this, Quartermaster Campbell assumed her duties, and, accompanied by her model from the Grand, sought out the Supply Depot. She returned with most superabundant rations, the male quartermaster apologising and puzzled ; for he could not understand how or

G

why they had got so much. Miss Campbell's
account was :

' An orderly asked me if I would like a side of
bacon, and when I said yes, he put it in the car.
And another said a case of peaches would be useful
and put it in. And some one else brought the
jam and the cheese, and they said a bag of tea
and another of sugar would not come amiss. And
just as we were leaving, a sergeant threw in two
hams.'

' So there it all is,' she ended gleefully.

On the following day, the 6th of November,
the hospital was ready for occupation ; the
plumber and gas-fitter were ejected, the pantry
became an operating theatre, the greenhouse was
converted into a linen room and packstore. In
the evening the ambulances met the trains, and
the large ward on the ground floor filled up.
Before very long all the beds were occupied, and
the Chief Surgeon and her two assistants were
kept busy with severe cases and heavy surgery.
The pressure of work continued until January ;
and both doctors and nurses had their hands full.
The place was small enough to be very personal,
and the relationship between the staff and the
men was a close one.

The women felt strangely near the Front, for

the men came down from the lines in a few hours, and their tales of the mud and wet in which they were standing almost up to their waists, the agony of frostbite, the terrible shortage of ammunition and the superiority of the German guns made pitiful hearing. The anxiety and strain of the severe cases was as nothing to the pathos of the slight cases who had to be sent straight back. As the day came nearer, their eyes would follow the Chief Surgeon round the ward, apprehensive of discharge ; and when at last the moment of farewell came, they were silent, for fear of losing their composure. A parcel of all the comforts possible was prepared for each one, and the hospital turned out to see them off, and some one would go with them to ' Base Details,' as the reporting station was called. But there was no getting over the horror of going back. Many of them, when they came out, had had no idea of what was before them ; and others were unfitted by temperament and by their former life for all they had to endure.

A Lancashire operative, no longer a young man, told how he had put his name to a paper.

' Missus she said I should, and so I did, but I never thought anything would coom of it.'

Then one day as he sat at dinner a military escort knocked at his door and called him out.

' But they coom for me,' he went on, ' at one
o'clock they coom, just as I was settin' down to
my dinner they coom, and took me outside, and the
orficer he said, " Now, A——, you 're soldier, and
if you desert, you will be shot," says he, and they
took me away. I had often heard tell of abroad
and I thought I would like to go, but I never
thought abroad was like this. Just a sea o' mood,
abroad is ! I don't want to coom abroad no more.'

It was very easy for friends to come over from
England, and many of them took advantage of
the opportunity. They did not come empty-
handed, and the hospital was supplied with games
and gramophones, and with abundance of such
things as water - beds and air - rings. Sir Alan
Anderson arrived with a car load of pheasants,
which were the last word in luxury. And work
depots were kind in sending linen and warm
clothing.

It was in this hospital that a suffragist friend
met and recognised a wounded policemen. She
claimed his acquaintance.

' I remember you,' she said. ' You arrested
me once in Whitehall.'

' I wouldn't have mentioned it, Miss,' he replied
with embarrassment. ' We 'll let byegones be
byegones.'

There was a constant stream of official visitors —colonels, inspectors and consultants—all of whom were more or less eager to pass men on— to send them to England or back to the line. The surgical work came in for a good deal of scrutiny ; for the R.A.M.C. were zealous about the turn-over, and went round every week or sometimes oftener, with the desire of emptying beds. Through constant observation, it was borne in upon these officers that the professional work and the organisation of the women were worthy of a wider opportunity ; and when the chance of saying a word of commendation came, that word was generously and freely said.

CHAPTER X

CLOSURE OF THE HOSPITAL IN THE HÔTEL CLARIDGE

EARLY in December trains of British sick and wounded were brought into Paris and the hospital on the Champs Élysées was filled to overflowing. In order to make additional accommodation, the large central hall had been closed in and furnished as a ward, and extra beds had been placed in the side wards.

The main problem, which became more pressing as the winter advanced, was how to procure enough coal to heat the huge building. The heating system was an extravagant one, for it was impossible to heat the hotel in sections, and if heat were raised for the ground floor, the whole of the seven stories had to participate, while the five great furnace boilers ate up the fuel with marvellous rapidity. It became necessary to introduce brazzeros into the wards. By this means the patients were kept fairly comfortable, although there were many objections to their use. A continual effort was required to secure enough fuel for cooking and for keeping the water hot, and neither M. Casanova nor M. Aubry nor M. Falcouz was successful in maintaining the supply.

Christmas found the hospital very full, and preparations for decorating the wards began unusually early. The British soldier had preconceived ideas with regard to paper chains, and thought that a blanket decorated with crude mottoes in cotton-wool and holly berries was the last word in mural decoration. The Poilu watched his operations in silence till his artistic soul rose within him, and snatching the chalk, with an impatient ' Tiens,' he too went down on the floor and sketched amazing pictures, directing with the voice of the master the colouring and embellishment of his designs.

In the end the walls were hung with aeroplanes, long guns, rising suns, statues to Liberty and Victory, mixed with British mottoes : ' Good Luck to the Women's Hospital Corps,' ' God Bless Mr. Davies,' and ' A Happy New Year to the Doctors ' ; while, overhead, paper chains of many hues were draped and the flags of all nations were prominently and abundantly displayed. In one ward every bedstead had the four Allied flags bound to each post, and in another a large dark coloured blanket displayed three battleships and a Union Jack, under which was traced 'The Flag of Freedom,' in letters of cotton-wool.

'Freedom!' said the *Médecin-en-Chef* to the Sister, with the treatment of militant women suffragists still fresh in her memory. 'Freedom! There is no freedom for women under that flag.'

The men were a little disappointed, for this was their great effort, and that it should fail to please, when all the rest of the decorations were commended, puzzled them. For some days before Christmas the wards were open to visitors, and crowds of people came to admire them. A sergeant taking a lady round paused before this masterpiece, and she too made the same comment.

'That's just what the doctor says, and we can't think what she means,' he exclaimed.

That night, when the doctor made her round, the word 'Freedom' had become 'England,' and as she looked at it with a comprehending smile growing on her face, a voice from the group round the brazzero said:

'We 're all for Votes for Women, Doctor.'

'Yes,' said another, 'even the Frenchies is for it.'

On Christmas Eve Mr. Bennett brought the choir boys from the Church to sing carols in the wards, and it was touching to see them grouped between the wards, wearing their white surplices and carrying coloured lanterns, which gleamed in the darkness. While the old melodies echoed through the hospital, the night nurses slipped from bed to bed, hanging socks on each one, and the final preparations for the next day's festivities were hastily completed behind the scenes.

At five o'clock on the festive morning the whole place awoke to the sound of laughter. Tin trumpets and jews' harps, tumbling pigs and false noses, evoked shouts of joy, reminiscent of nursery life. The spirit of Christmas descended on the hospital and pain and care were forgotten.

M. Casanova had found splendid turkeys and sausages, and plum puddings had been sent from England. Mr. Davies had procured beer and there was port wine for the King's health. Long tables were set for those who were up, and the beds of those who were not up were collected in the large ward. Only one officer, Lieut. Vogel, was in the hospital that day, and he gave the French toasts, and joined in all the fun with great delight. The procession of puddings was hailed with acclamation. The toasts were drunk and the crackers pulled with energy and much noise. Every one feasted and made merry. Later there was an entertainment in the big hall, to which many guests had been invited, including all the Belgians from the seventh story.

The concert began, with a sergeant in the chair, and was going well, when Colonel S—— and his quartermaster and several sergeants arrived to distribute Princess Mary's gifts to the men. Some weeks before, a nominal roll of men who would be in hospital had been required, and the hospital was hardly to blame if the roll had altered since that date. At the last moment two new rolls had to be made, one for smokers and one for non-smokers, and this task had been much complicated by a desire on the part of many recipients to change over from one roll to the other. The colonel arrived without warning, and was embarrassed to find himself on a platform, facing a large crowd of people. In consequence, he lost his place on the roll and made mistakes about the names, and confused the smokers and non-smokers ; but in the end he got through the distribution, and merry-making was resumed.

The *chef-d'œuvre* was the Pantomime, arranged by the staff. Mr. Davies was consulted about an abridged version of ' Red Riding Hood,' and was so horrified by the amateurish suggestions that he refused to write it. He said his reputation

would never survive it ; so, if it was written at
all, Baroness Geysa de Braunecker and Dr. Cuthbert wrote it, or threw it together ; for the con-
struction left much to be desired. The actors
(having no reputations) were not at all nervous,
and they appointed Mr. Davies stage manager
and instructed him to take one cue and pass a
cow's head through the screen. Divided between
laughter and nervousness, he forgot his cue about
Maud, the cow ; and the performer called so
frequently for Maud that the room took it up and
shouted for Maud, until, with a shaking hand, a
large pasteboard cow's head was pushed through.
The hall became uproarious over the flight of
the grandmother pursued by the wolf, and many
hands were stretched out to catch the wolf and
give the old lady a chance. The day ended, as it
had begun, with laughter and cheers. And as
night fell there was a quiet hour, smoking in the
wards and talking it over. The men said that
they had never known such a Christmas : it was
something to tell in the trenches, something to
write home—a memory treasured by patients and
staff alike.

The Pantomime had inspired the men to give
dramatic entertainments on their own account,
and almost every evening the staff enjoyed seeing

a play arranged and rehearsed by the patients, which was often full of humour and of pathos. One, entitled ' The Murder of Mr. Smith,' in which a judge was represented who wore a cotton-wool wig and who constantly roared out ' Silence in Court ! ' ; and another, ' The Deserter,' stand out in the memory of those who saw them. The latter was a pathetic little drama. The officers at the Court Martial were faithfully portrayed : the bullying sergeant-major, the bouncing lieu- tenant, the courageous accused, were all recog- nisable types. And the death sentence, carried out on the stage, moved one strangely. The acting was simple and intelligent, and the theme a very living one to those men in those days. After the play there would be music and songs, with the Baroness at the piano and Mrs. Henley leading and conducting from the steps.

' My ! this is a place ! ' a sergeant from a neighbouring hospital said to Mrs. Henley. He had come with a message from Colonel S—— and had found his way into the hall one evening. ' This is a place ! You would be pleased if you heard how they are all talking about you.'

The patients, too, appreciated the place and wrote glowing accounts of its grandeur and its pleasures to friends at home.

'I'd be happy,' wrote a wife, 'if you was stopping there till the war was over.'

And many messages of thanks reached the Sisters from mothers in England. Photographs of babies and little boys in velveteen suits arrived by post, so that the doctors might see what fine children they had. And the Poilus were always proud if opportunity allowed them to introduce Madame. One of the older men, who was confined to bed with rheumatism, consulted the doctor as to the best way of sending a registered parcel to his wife.

'It will be vallyble furs,' he said.

And the doctor thought he must have been looting, until it transpired that he wished to send her the goat-skin coat which had been issued for his own use.

'I don't seem to fancy it for myself,' he said, 'but the Missus would look proper in it.'

'They pay you the compliment of not wishing to leave,' said a general after his round of inspection. And indeed it was with very mixed feelings that men ready for evacuation left the hospital, even though evacuation meant going straight to England. There were many handshakings, promises 'not to forget you,' grateful thanks and not

uncommonly tears in the eyes of the men as they
drove away, making the Champs Élysées resound
to the strains of ' Auld Lang Syne.'

As the weather grew colder, all M. Casanova's
efforts to procure coal were unavailing, and very
often there was not enough to maintain the supply
of hot water. This was the case on one occasion
when notice was received that eighty patients
were arriving, and no hot baths were available ;
and much time and labour was spent in preparing
gallons of hot water for toilet purposes over the gas
rings. When the wards were very cold, the men
were kept in bed with hot bottles and blankets ;
but obviously this plan could not be continued
indefinitely, and as no help was forthcoming from
' l'intendance militaire,' the question of closing
the hospital had to be considered. The French
Red Cross had other hospitals in Paris, and many
of these had not yet been opened. They were
unwilling to close ' Claridge's,' which had been
very useful to both French and British troops ;
but they were helpless over the matter of fuel,
and during the winter months the pressure of
work was not very great. They regarded the
hospital as their ' meilleure installation.' It had
been a great interest and a great revelation not

only to the officials of the Red Cross but to many people outside it, and they were reluctant to part with it. In addition, they began to have some difficulty with M. Casanova, and it was understood that he had offered the building without the authority of his Board of Directors, and that the presence of the hospital in the Hôtel was embarrassing to him.

British officials were equally unwilling to lose the hospital. One wrote : ' You have set a standard which is quite unknown even among auxiliary hospitals.' And another said : ' It would be a misfortune if you were to leave. You are such a good example of what a hospital ought to be.'

Nevertheless, it was decided in conference between M. Pérouse, M. Falcouz and Dr. Flora Murray that, in view of the circumstances, the hospital should be closed. The decision was reached after much consideration, and with deep regret the staff turned to the task of evacuation and packing.

The hospital closed on the 18th of January 1915. The doctors and nurses proceeded to Wimereux to join forces with the rest of the Corps, bearing with them the good wishes and kind farewells of their many friends in Paris.

The hospital in the Hôtel Claridge was the first effort of the Women's Hospital Corps. It brought help to the wounded at a time when such help was greatly needed. It gave women doctors an opportunity of showing their capacity for surgery under war conditions. It was one of the outstanding pieces of work done by women in those first months of war, and it was a great success.

CHAPTER XI

THE CORPS IS OFFERED A HOSPITAL IN LONDON

THE hospital at Wimereux was lighter than it had been for many weeks, for the winter weather had caused a lull in the fighting. In February it was evident that the constant rains and the state of the ground at the Front would make any advance impossible for weeks to come. The patients coming down to the base were chiefly medical cases or had slight injuries, which made their early transfer to England possible ; and the work assumed more and more the character of a clearing station.

In conversation with the Assistant Director of Medical Services, it was learnt that fifty thousand additional hospital beds were to be set up in England that spring, and that the supply of doctors—especially of doctors who could organise —was far short of the Army's requirements. The organisers had now to consider whether the Corps could be of greater service in England than in France. General W——, with whom this

H

question was discussed, stated that the pressure
of work would probably lie in England, and that
the services of the Women's Hospital Corps
would certainly be acceptable there.

'You must not give up military work,' he said
to Dr. Garrett Anderson and Dr. Flora Murray.
And with real kindness he sent a despatch to the
Director General about their work, and advised
them to ask for an interview with him at the
War Office.

Preceded by General W—'s despatch and their
letter enclosing various introductions and asking
for an appointment, Dr. Garrett Anderson and
Dr. Flora Murray arrived in London. Here
rumour met them with reports of the intentions
of the Director General and of his favourable
disposition towards them, and it was with a not
unnatural thrill of anticipation that they entered
the War Office.

Surgeon-General Sir Alfred Keogh, G.C.V.O.,
G.C.B., opened the interview by saying that he
had heard a great deal about their hospitals,
that he had heard nothing but good, and that
he expected them to manage a larger formation
than a hundred beds.

'Who is running you ? ' he asked.

'Nobody. We run ourselves.'

' Yes ! but who is behind you ?   What lady ? '

' There is no lady.'

' Who gets your money ? '

' We get it ourselves.'

' Well, but who is your committee ?

' We are the committee.'

' Ah then,' he said, with a twinkling eye, ' then we can talk.'

It was a very pleasant talk, in the course of which the Director General said that he required large units, for small ones were no good to him at that time. And he arranged to take the women doctors on ' in the usual way ' and to give them charge of a hospital of five hundred or a thousand beds. The staff was to consist of women, with as few R.A.M.C. men as possible. The task of finding doctors and nurses was to rest with the organisers. In the meantime, he asked them to close the hospital in France and to bring the Unit over to London.

Dr. Garrett Anderson and Dr. Flora Murray returned to France next day, and the business of closing the hospital in the Château Mauricien began at once. A number of the nursing sisters who had done arduous and devoted work in Paris and Wimereux expressed their intention of joining the Corps in its new hospital, and were

consequently hurried off to England, so that
they might have a rest and recuperate before the
next demand was made upon their health and
energy. The quartermaster and orderlies, full
of delightful enthusiasm for the future, made
short work of the packing and all the winding up
of affairs. A large part of the equipment, especially such things as coloured blankets, linen and
extras which add to the comfort of wards, were
reserved for use in London. The rest was taken
over by the Ordnance, to the annoyance of the
quartermaster who had to receive it, because
it was not according to the scheduled pattern.

Dr. Garrett Anderson and Dr. Flora Murray
took an early opportunity of calling upon the
Assistant Director of Medical Services, who
greeted them with his usual kindness.

' Come and tell us how you got on with the
Director General—what is he going to give you ? '
he asked.

' He is going to put us in charge of a hospital
of five hundred and twenty beds in London,'
replied Dr. Garrett Anderson.

' Good God ! he isn't ? ' gasped the colonel,
falling back in his chair with surprise. Then,
recovering from his astonishment, he added
kindly :

' Well, when I think of it, I expect you 'll be able to do it.'

His congratulations and advice were most friendly.

' You must insist upon one thing,' he said. ' They must give you good warrant officers. Otherwise you 'll have awful trouble with your discipline.'

' We never have had any trouble,' said Dr. Flora Murray.

' I know you haven't,' he answered. ' We have often spoken of it, and wondered how you managed ; for you have never come to us for help. But now it will be different. You 've always been ladies ; now you 'll both be colonels, and you 'll see what a difference it makes.'

There remained only the final arrangements to be made. The requisitioned articles were returned and the house was handed over to the *maire*, who remarked regretfully that he had never made so little out of any one before ! The farewell calls were paid, a farewell dinner was given, and the Belgian staff was paid off and disposed elsewhere.

On the day when they were ready to cross the morning boat was not running ; for the Germans had just announced their submarine campaign in the Channel. The night boat, however, was sailing ; and quite late, with the connivance of the purser, the little party, which included Dr. Garrett Anderson, Dr. Flora Murray and two others, managed to get on board, and lay very low in a corner. But at 11.30 the Transport Officer came stamping through the saloons, shouting that all civilians and ladies were to go ashore, and they were hastily turned out on to the muddy quay in the pouring rain. After a delay of forty-eight hours places on board a hospital ship were courteously placed at their disposal, and they finally arrived at Dover on the 19th of February 1915.

On reaching London they learnt that Sir Alfred Keogh had made public his intentions with regard to the future of the Women's Hospital Corps the day before. Speaking at a meeting at Sunderland House, in favour of the extension of the London School of Medicine for Women, on the 18th of February 1915, he said :

' He had received numbers of unsolicited letters from Paris and Boulogne, which stated that the work of women doctors at the Front was beyond all praise ; it was an example of how such work ought to be done. So impressed had he been that he had asked two of the staff from Paris and Boulogne to come here and do bigger work. He had asked them to take charge of a hospital of 500 beds and, if they pleased, of a hospital of 1000 beds. (Cheers).'—*The Times*, 19th February 1915.

The audience, which was composed largely of people interested in the development of the work of medical women, received this announcement with every sign of pleasure and approbation. Sir Alfred Keogh was cordially congratulated by the other speakers upon the wisdom and courage with which he had made himself responsible for an innovation of such magnitude and importance. His action was destined to lead subsequently to that extensive development of Women's Services which proved so valuable and so necessary in the conduct of the war.

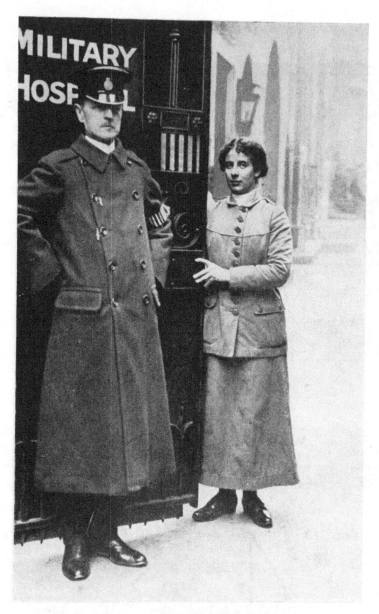

THE GATE OF THE MILITARY HOSPITAL, ENDELL STREET, AND
THE TRANSPORT OFFICER—MISS M. E. HODGSON

(Page 122)

(Photo, Alfieri)

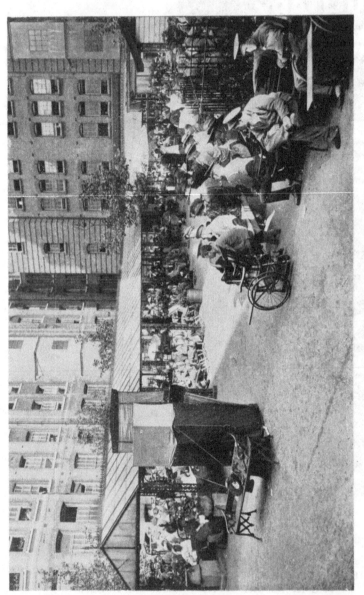

AN AUGUST BANK HOLIDAY

(Photo, Alfieri)

(Page 123)

PART II

THE WOMEN'S HOSPITAL CORPS IN LONDON

CHAPTER I

ORGANISATION OF THE MILITARY HOSPITAL
ENDELL STREET

THE old workhouse of St. Giles, Bloomsbury, had
been taken over by the War Office for hospital
purposes, and it was there that the Director
General decided to station the Women's Hospital
Corps.

The group of buildings rises, grey and sombre-
looking, at the upper end of Endell Street, on
ground which was granted by Queen Matilda for
a lepers' hospital. It abuts on Shorts Gardens,
where the leper colony lingered long after Henry
VIII. had absorbed the original foundation. Some
months before the war, the Guardians had evacuated these premises for grander and more com-
modious quarters elsewhere, and during 1914
the buildings had been occupied by Belgian
refugees. In the spring of 1915 an army of
workmen took possession, and the work of reno-
vating and adapting them for a hospital was
already advancing. A narrow entrance, partially
hidden by Christ's Church, led into a square,

formed by three large hospital blocks, the church
and a long administrative building. A glass-
covered passage ran down the centre of the square
and across to either block. It was fenced in
with high iron railings, and the free space on
either side was divided by more railings into
little pens. The little pens had padlocked gates
and were labelled : ' Old Males,' ' Young Males,'
' Old Females,' ' Young Females ; ' and it was
in these cages that the inmates of the workhouse
had sought fresh air and recreation. There was a
little gate office next to the mortuary, where a
set of pigeon holes, constructed out of slate slabs,
was designed to receive coffins, and where the
gas meter took up most of the room. Behind
the main buildings were the children's home—
modern and well built—and the Guardians' offices,
opening on to Broad Street. Part of the administrative block bore the date 1727, and St. Giles
was said to have been the workhouse described
by Dickens in *Oliver Twist*. A long room, with
a fireplace at either end, still exists in the oldest
part, where Oliver is supposed to have been
interviewed by the Guardians ; and the cellars
or basements under this section of the building
are of the most ancient and grimy description.
The hospital blocks were five stories high, with

good air space and large wards. There were windows on both sides of these wards, and more sunshine and fresh air were available than was expected in that locality. The warehouses next door were in the hands of the A.S.C.M.T., and all round lay the teeming, crowded streets of Soho and Drury Lane.

Extensive structural alterations were necessary. Lifts capable of carrying stretchers were put in ; the sanitation was renewed, and electric light and modern cooking apparatus were installed. The building was cleaned and painted throughout, but there was an extraordinary amount of old furniture and disused apparatus which the Guardians had left behind, and the presence of piles of lumber was embarrassing. The fittings of padded rooms and curious pieces of furniture, designed to restrain the insane, came out of the lunacy block ; antique baths and obsolete drain-pipes were cast out by the builders, and in their place ward kitchens and bathrooms were arranged on every floor ; and operating theatres, X-ray room, laboratories, dispensaries and store-rooms were completed.

Acting upon instructions from the Director General, Dr. Garrett Anderson and Dr. Flora Murray, since their return, had been engaged in finding staff and in drawing up a scheme for the future establishment. Their final destination was not decided until early in March, when they were summoned to the War Office to discuss the suitability of Endell Street. On the way to keep their appointment, they stepped inside the gate and surveyed with a rapid glance the lie of the buildings and the piles of rubbish and dirt massed among the iron railings in the square. They saw enough to enable them to say that it would do, before the gate-keeper turned them out as being unauthorised persons upon government premises.

The feeling of the Army Medical Department towards women doctors could be gauged by the atmosphere in the various offices with which business had to be done. In one there was disapproval ; in another curiosity and amusement ; in a third obstinate hostility, which was not dissipated by an unassuming manner. But in the Director General's own office a most cordial desire to assist was met with, and nothing was left undone to that end. He himself put the doctors in touch with a young major in the department, instructing him to give them every possible assistance and telling them to go to him in any difficulty. Further, he sent them to see the Deputy Director of Medical Services for the

London District, and so launched them on the War Office tide.

The young major — who shortly became a colonel—was obviously nervous of being seen in such company, and in the manner of a sheepish schoolboy secluded them in his own little den. There the limit of his knowledge was soon reached, but he was able to indicate the rooms of several colonels who ought to be seen. Fearful of making a public appearance in the corridors again, he telephoned through to these gentlemen, and with relief despatched the ladies, under the guidance of an N.C.O. A few days later, when he was approached with regard to some small difficulty, he said that he knew nothing about hospitals and that it was no good coming to him— a plain truth which was already becoming apparent both where he and other officers were concerned.

By the light of experience gained in the years which followed, the doctors realised how much these War Office officials could and should have done to help them in those early days, and how they did as little as possible. Thus they created on the minds of these women an impression, which may or may not have been correct, of incompetence and want of intelligence. Advice and assistance were withheld, lest the officer who

gave it might in some way become responsible
for the women's affairs; and in addition, their
path was often obstructed. It was not understood at the time that obstruction was due to
hostility : it was taken for stupidity, or the way
in which things were done at the War Office ;
and after two or three fruitless visits to the branch
offices of the Army Medical Department no
further time was wasted on these gentlemen.
Other sources of information or other ways of
getting things through were discovered.

The Director General had arranged for the
senior medical officers and the quartermaster to
take a course of instruction in administration
under the Officer-in-Charge of the Queen Alexandra
Military Hospital, Millbank ; and this officer and
his staff showed them much kindness and gave
them, with many hints as to procedure, a valuable
insight into the working of a well-directed military
hospital.

In due course an appointment was made with
the officer then in charge of the alterations at
Endell Street, in order that he might take the
doctors round the premises and give them information which would enable them to complete
their scheme of establishment.

Two officers, a quartermaster, an N.C.O. and

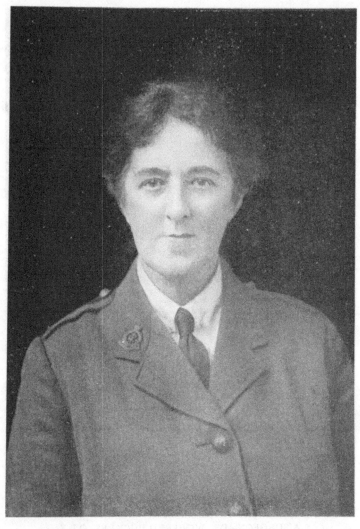

THE OPHTHALMIC SURGEON—DR. AMY SHEPPARD, O.B.E.

(Page 134)

(*Photo, Russell*)

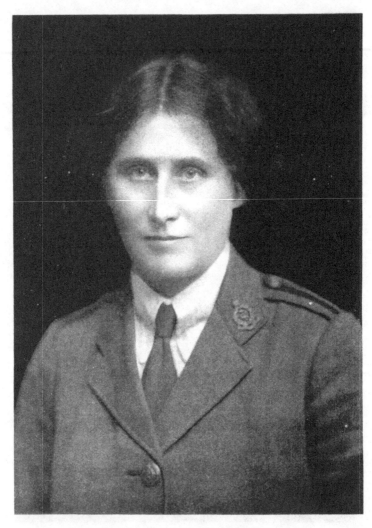

A SURGEON—DR. WINIFRED BUCKLEY, O.B.E

(Page 135)

(*Photo, A. Basil*)

six privates—R.A.M.C.—were living in the buildings and were engaged in making preparations; but
owing to the state of the works and the mess in
the place, they were—so the colonel said—' marking time.' The colonel was what the soldiers
call ' a real R.A.M.C. colonel.' The idea of women
doctors in a military hospital was very distasteful
to him. The proposal filled him with disgust
and apprehension, and he was firmly convinced
it was not feasible.

' Good God ! *Women* !' he ejaculated. ' God
bless my soul, *Women* !'

He writhed on his chair and, perspiring heavily,
spoke for an hour (with frequent ejaculations
about ' Women !') in an endeavour to prove
that the idea was ridiculous and impossible in
any hospital, but especially so in that particular
one. Being reminded that the matter had been
settled and that the doctors desired to go over the
buildings, he questioned the sanity of the War
Office, and finding himself unable to stay any
longer in the vicinity of such ' indelicate females,'
he firmly declared that he was going out, and he
marched off, exclaiming :

' Oh, good God ! what difficulties you will have.'

The second officer followed him silently. The
quartermaster-sergeant, who had been present all

the time, pretended that he did not know his way round the building, so Dr. Garrett Anderson and Dr. Flora Murray set out alone on a tour of inspection. From what they saw they concluded that, if the hospital were to open in May, 'marking time' must cease, and they therefore wrote to the Director General, requesting that they might be put in charge at once. By return of post came their instructions, and on the 22nd of March 1915 the Military Hospital, Endell Street, was handed over to them by the chastened and protesting colonel. There remained, to superintend the structural alterations, a captain in the R.E. and the contractor's clerk of works, Mr. Cook. The latter was a civilian and a real patriot. He was destined to become a great ally and, incidentally, a staunch feminist. The rapid progress made in the work was due to his energy and devotion.

The premises were encumbered by the presence of much worn-out and obsolete furniture—the discarded property of the Guardians. A certain portion of it could be made use of, and this was picked out and cleaned for the wards or the quarters of the staff; but a great deal of it was useless, and urgent requests were made for its immediate removal. It included several hundred old flock mattresses; and these, by direction of the above-mentioned colonel, had been stored in the laundry. This was a fine, large room, and it was filled up to the door with dirty and somewhat damp bedding. The danger of heating was obvious, and in addition the laundry itself was the only available place for a linen store. The colonel and the R.E. captain had decided that the hospital would not require this room, and the cleaning of it had been cut out of the estimates. As an alternative they suggested that linen, bedding and clothing for six hundred men should be kept in a little basement store. After much opposition and delay, it was sanctioned that the laundry should be used, and renewed efforts were made to induce the Guardians to remove their material. More than one visit was made to the Clerk of the Guardians before the name of the official who was really responsible was elicited. It slipped out quite inadvertently in conversation one morning. The Clerk had no sooner said it than he regretted it, for he was promptly required to telephone and see if this gentleman was available.

It was Saturday morning and though he was in his office, he was leaving early to catch a train. As the doctors hastily left the room, they heard the Clerk, in accents of dismay, saying down the

telephone, 'They have started!' Arrived at
the other office, it was clear that the hall-porter
and secretaries were anxious to prevent an interview with their chief; but the doctors, instead
of sitting down in the waiting-room with a closed
door, as they were invited to do, followed closely
on the heels of the distressed porter and were
so close behind him that they could not be refused entrance to the office and the presence
of the Chairman. He had his hat on, his bag in
his hand, and in another second he would have
been gone.

'I have a train to catch,' he cried.

'We won't keep you a moment: just give
orders to have all that furniture and bedding
removed.'

'I will attend to it on Monday, certainly.'

'Monday is too late. A telephone message
now, please.'

He hesitated, looked at them standing between
him and the door, laughed and capitulated.

'All right, ring them up,' he said to his secretary, and fled to catch his train. But the women
remained to hear the order sent through.

By the end of the month Dr. Garrett Anderson
and Dr. Flora Murray had moved into the quarters
at Endell Street, which they continued to occupy

until April 1919. And the work of preparation was progressing rapidly. Under Mr. Cook's influence, the workmen gave up their Easter holiday, and every one pressed forward eagerly. Indents were drawn up and sent in for the furniture and medical stores required, and gradually the supplies were delivered. Several years later, Major B—— told Dr. Flora Murray with what interest the first indents from Endell Street had been scanned at the Horse Guards, and how surprising it had been to find that they were right.

The furniture arrived before the lifts were ready and in quantities which the small R.A.M.C. contingent could not deal with. Fatigue parties, therefore, from the various regiments stationed in London were obtained, and the furniture and equipment were distributed through the buildings.

At this stage, a very kind old gentleman—not in uniform—came into the square and inquired how we were getting on. He said that he was the Officer in Charge of Barracks, and that the indents for furniture, linen, etc., went through his office. In conversation he stated that he was in his eightieth year, and he showed a friendly interest in the plans for the hospital. He had two daughters who were both suffragists.

' One,' he said, ' belongs to a most respectable

society,' then dropping his voice, 'but the other
—she goes with Mrs. Pankhurst's lot.'

Perhaps his hearers, who had also gone with
'Mrs. Pankhurst's lot' in the suffrage days, did
not look as shocked as he expected ; for he added
kindly :

'I daresay you may not have heard of Mrs.
Pankhurst.'

One morning, as he watched a fatigue party
fall in in the square, he asked :

'Now, do you get any work out of these fellows ? '

'Yes,' answered Dr. Garrett Anderson, 'there
is a woman placed at the bottom of the stairs to
send them up, and another at the top to send
them down again, and they get quite a lot done.'

'Poor fellows, poor fellows,' said the major.
'Very energetic ladies ! Oh ! we are not accustomed to that in the Army.'

The Corps required to be largely supplemented
to enable it to cope with the work before it, but
fortunately it was able to fall back upon a number
of its original members, and these formed the
nucleus of the new staff. Dr. Woodcock became
the physician to the hospital. Dr. Gertrude
Gazdar and Dr. Rosalie Jobson, who had worked
in France, accepted posts as assistant surgeons.
Dr. Amy Sheppard, O.B.E., was appointed oph-

thalmic surgeon; Dr. Helen Chambers, C.B.E., pathologist; Dr. Eva Handley-Read, dental surgeon; and Dr. E. M. Magill, O.B.E., radiologist (in 1916); while Dr. Winifred Buckley, O.B.E., who served from the opening of the hospital to its closure, and three other doctors, completed the surgical staff. Dr. Louisa Garrett Anderson, C.B.E., was the Chief Surgeon, and the administrative work, with title of 'Doctor-in-Charge,' fell to Dr. Flora Murray, C.B.E.

Miss Hale, R.R.C., who was then matron of the Elizabeth Garrett Anderson Hospital and a member of the Territorial Force Nursing Service, was working at the 1st London General Hospital at the time. Dr. Flora Murray represented to Sir Alfred Keogh that she was the right person to take up the work of matron, and by his wish, and with the cordial consent of Dame Sidney Browne, D.B.E., R.R.C., Matron-in-Chief, Territorial Force Nursing Service, she was seconded for service under the War Office. She held the office of matron with success from April 1915 till October 1919. Some of the Sisters from the French hospitals, Miss Breen, Miss Pearson, Mrs. Lawrence, R.R.C., Miss Clemow, R.R.C., and Miss Belton, continued as members of the Corps. The schedule of establishment sanctioned only thirty-six trained nurses for the entire hospital. Words cannot measure or describe the value of their service to the sick and wounded. Some of them, including Sister May, Sister Beales and Sister Moore remained from the opening date until its closure. They worked at high pressure, often under difficulties, and with untrained subordinates, while surgeons and patients learnt to rely more and more upon their constant care and devotion.

Quartermaster Campbell expanded her staff to meet requirements, and the former orderlies, Miss M. E. Hodgson and Miss Isabel Lowe, were called up early to help in organising. A hundred picked young women joined up as orderlies, some for nursing and some for administrative work ; while the clerical section was organised by Miss Jarvis, who had also served with the Corps in France, and by Miss Esther Hatten. The R.A.M.C. detachment numbered one N.C.O. and twenty men, fourteen of whom were later replaced by women. Thus a staff of approximately one hundred and eighty persons was ready when the hospital opened in May.

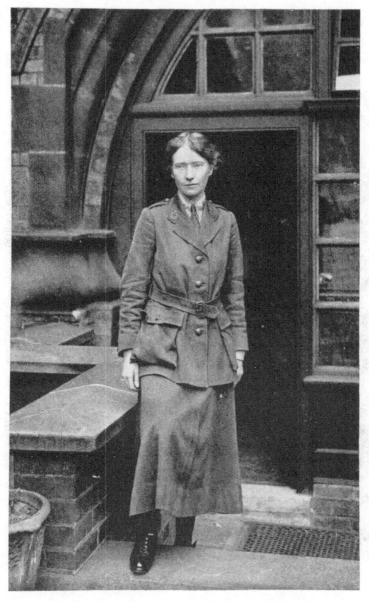

THE PATHOLOGIST—DR. HELEN CHAMBERS, C.B.E.

(Page 138)

(*Photo, Reginald Haines*)

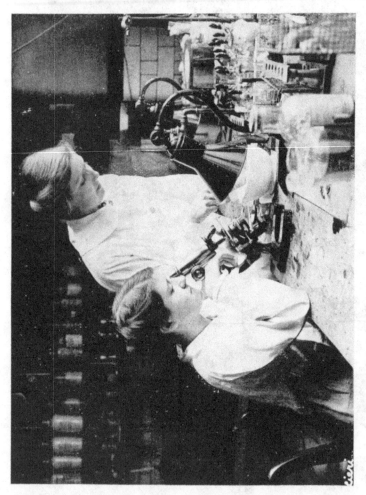

SEARCHING FOR PROTOZOA IN THE LABORATORY

(Page 139)

CHAPTER II

FIRST DAYS OF THE MILITARY HOSPITAL
ENDELL STREET

THE hospital was designed to accommodate five hundred and twenty cases, but it had not been open long before orders were received to put up as many extra beds as possible ; and from 1916 onwards the number of beds was five hundred and seventy - three. Several auxiliary V.A.D. hospitals were attached to it at a later date, supplying another hundred and fifty beds. At times of pressure, when billeting of convalescent men was allowed, the numbers on the register approximated to eight hundred. Once the extra beds went up, they were not taken down again, and it was not until the summer of 1919 that any reduction was made.

There were seventeen wards, of which the three smaller ones in the south block were reserved for severe cases. They all had ample window space, and though the beds were closer than is usual or desirable in civilian hospitals, there was plenty of fresh air and light. The chilly whitewashed walls and gloomy brown blankets of Army hospitals seen in France were not forgotten, and great trouble was taken to make the Endell Street Hospital look gay and comfortable. Every ward had its flowers and its red and blue or scarlet blankets to give it colour, and its table and screen covers to give it an air of comfort. The electric lighting, as carried out by the R.E. in spite of demonstration and remonstrance, was hopeless ; with only three or four single drop lights in the centre of a ward for thirty or forty men, no one in bed could see to read or play cards. An application for standard lights produced, after long correspondence and delay, only the scheduled number of thirty ; and the lighting was not arranged satisfactorily until the St. Leonard's School stepped in and sent one hundred and eighty standards for ward use. This generous gift made every one comfortable, and the necessity for drafting report after report, to support applications for more than the scheduled number of lamps, ceased.

The lifts were large enough to carry beds, and in fine weather it was usual to find rows of beds and wheel chairs in the square, which had been cleared of all the impedimenta and railings belonging to its workhouse past, and which made a

pleasant general meeting ground. A large recreation room was available for wet days. At
one end there was a small green-room and stage,
which the Corps out of its own funds supplied
with electric batons and curtains. The drop
curtain was of saxe blue, with monogram ' W.H.C.'
in black and orange, and the motto of the Corps,
' Deeds not Words,' was proudly mounted above
the proscenium. This room also housed the
library and billiard table.

The patients' dining room was a somewhat
gloomy place on the ground floor in the neighbourhood of the kitchen ; but only the very
convalescent descended to it at midday and spent
there the few minutes which a soldier man re-
quires for consuming a hearty meal. The more
experienced Sisters had an ineradicable objection
to not knowing what and how ' their men ' ate,
and persistently discountenanced the dining-hall.

On the ground floor of the south block the large
windows of the pathological laboratory and the
dispensary afforded those who worked inside a
fine view of the square and prevented them
from feeling cut off or isolated from the general
life of the place. On the top were found two
operating rooms and the X-ray room with its
appurtenances, as well as accommodation for the

dental surgeon. The ophthalmic surgeon worked up there too, in default of better quarters, adapting a passage and a corner of the dark room for the needs of her patients. In a building where there was not a corner to spare, and where people were constantly asking for ' a room of my own,' her uncomplaining consideration was much appreciated.

In every spare corner of the basements and ground floors, offices and store - rooms were crowded in. Above the quartermaster's office and steward's stores, three floors of cubicles were arranged as sleeping quarters for women orderlies ; and for some unknown reason this part of the building was called the ' Barracks.' The Children's Home housed the nursing sisters, and the Barracks and Guardians' Offices were full to overflowing with girls. The old Receiving House near the gate was occupied by the R.A.M.C. The Master's house, which had been built so as to command a good view of the square, provided offices and doctors' room on the first floor and living rooms above for the resident doctors, the orderly officer, the matron and several other people. Every corner was occupied, and as the work or the needs of the hospital expanded, it was a puzzle to find room. As the years went on, it became necessary for additional quarters to be found outside for the nursing staff, and two houses in the neighbourhood were eventually rented and adapted for the use of the hospital. It is noteworthy that although the first report and request for further accommodation described this need as ' very pressing,' it took an entire year to get the first of these houses passed by the military authorities and the necessary business completed for opening it.

In naming the wards, it was convenient to follow the alphabetical order, and in the desire to call them after women the names of saints, with a few others, were chosen. Thus Ward ' A ' was known as ' St. Anne.' ' St. Barbara ' and ' St. Catherine ' followed ; and, with one or two omissions, the sequence continued down to ' St. Veronica.' ' St. Ursula,' the patron saint of young women, was included, and in order to cover the letter ' O,' ' St. Onorio ' was invoked. She was afterwards found to be, not very appropriately, the patron saint of wet-nurses ! But she served her ward well, for it was one of the happiest in the hospital. ' St. Mary ' was unfortunate, and the ward never had very good luck until her name was changed to ' St. Margaret.' Rachel, in those tragic days of war, could not be omitted. Hilde-

garde, the famous medicine woman of the third
century, and the martyred St. Felicitas were
grouped with St. Geneviève of Paris and St. Isa-
bella of Spain. The idea was picturesque, and
the nomenclature pleased the staff, if it did not
appeal much to the men. A bare little room in
the basement was entitled the ' Johnny Walker
Ward,' and was used as a place of recovery by
his patrons and slaves.

Early in May the first return of available beds
was made ; for two blocks were ready for occupation and the third was nearly so. The delivery
of certain things, such as dinner tins, wagons
and knives and forks, was delayed, and promised
to be delayed for months. With activity increasing in France, the opening of the hospital
could not be postponed for such trifles, and the
resourceful quartermaster arranged to hire what
was needful for a month. The staff was called
up and settled down in its quarters ; the rows of
beds were got ready ; the stock bottles and cupboards were filled ; the instruments and apparatus
were issued on charge to the Sisters ; the kitchen
plant was in order. Though not yet completely
equipped, it was possible to inform Headquarters
that Endell Street was ready to open.

The Army way of opening a hospital is to

transfer to it convalescent cases from other hospitals. When asked at a later date why this custom prevailed, since it did not make things easier for the receiving hospital, a senior officer said that there was nothing to recommend the custom, but that that was the way they did it. In every hospital there were cases which, for some reason or another, the staff was more or less glad to pass on ; and an order to transfer twenty-five or fifty walking cases meant that the troublesome, the idle, the grousing, or those who were unsatisfactory for some reason, were collected and moved on. On the 12th of May 1915 Endell Street received a hundred convalescent cases from various hospitals in the London District. That night, the convoys from France began to arrive, and a letter written on the 14th to hasten the supply of knives and forks states that on that date there were two hundred and forty-six men in the hospital. It was open just as a spell of heavy fighting began, and within a week all its beds were available and all were full.

The first month was a difficult one. The work poured into the hospital, making new and heavy demands upon every one. Equipment was short, and the women had everything to learn and no one to advise or help them. They had to find things out for themselves, and some months later much time was spent in correcting, by the light of experience, entries in registers and returns which had been incorrectly made in those early days. Gradually order was evolved. The women adapted themselves to the conditions, and the wheels of the establishment went round more easily each week. The strain of those first days was severe ; the staff was weary in mind and body ; but the general eagerness to make things go right triumphed, and the organisation developed and established itself.

It soon became evident that Endell Street was a favourably situated hospital, and that it would not lack for work. It was near to the railway stations, and through all the years that followed its beds were kept very full and the proportion of cot cases—as against sitting cases—coming into its wards was a high one. It had a busy casualty room, too, where men from neighbouring stations reported sick in the mornings, and into which men on leave, or men absent without leave, would wander for more or less severe ailments. Men suffering from accidents or fits or drunkenness were liable to arrive in ambulances at all hours of the day and night, and more serious cases, from billets, from hotels or from

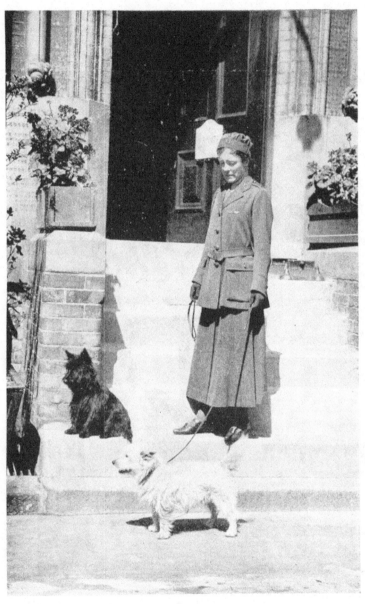

THE CHIEF SURGEON WITH GARRETT AND WILLIAM

(Page 148)

(Photo, Reginald Haines)

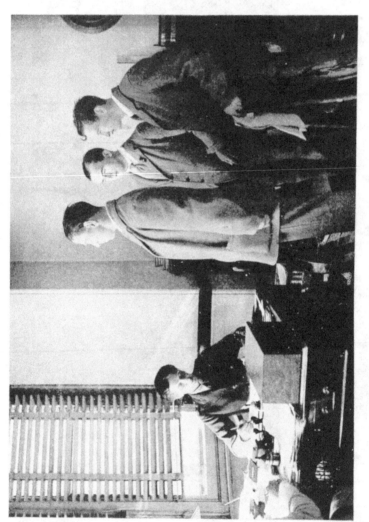

THE DOCTOR-IN-CHARGE SEES MEN IN HER OFFICE

(Page 149)

the St. Albans military district were constantly received there. In 1917 to 1919 numbers of pensioners came for treatment, and hundreds of men were examined and certified before demobilisation, or else attended after demobilisation to have the Army form relating to disabilities and assessments made up. The average number of attendances in the casualty room totalled not less than five thousand each year.

Twice, perhaps, a lull occurred in the convoys coming from overseas, and the return of empty beds rose to two hundred or so. The nursing staff would begin to complain of being slack, but such periods of quiet were followed by rushes of work, when two or three or four convoys would arrive in twenty-four hours, and every effort had to be made to discharge or transfer convalescents and make room for new-comers. As a rule, at busy times every bed emptied during the day was filled at night. On one such night, when four beds were returned, four fractured spines were sent in a few hours later.

A big bell hung in the square, and the arrival of a convoy was notified to the staff by two blows on it. This brought out those whose duty it was to assist in taking in. Doctors, women stretcher-bearers and R.A.M.C. assembled with-

out delay; for it was necessary to hasten and let
the ambulances get back to the station for a
second journey. The staff of men orderlies being
small, the women were all trained as bearers.
The men would unload the stretcher and hold
it, while women stepped between the handles
and carried it to the lift and so to the bedside.
Stretcher bearing was a popular occupation, and
if the bell rang during the day, volunteers would
run out of the stores and offices and laboratories
and fall in with the R.A.M.C. The man on the
stretcher was often speechless with astonishment
when he realised that two ' flappers ' were carrying him; but they were very steady, gentle
bearers, and earned high praise for the way in
which they performed their duties.

Out of twenty-six thousand patients who passed
through the wards, the greater number were
British, with a fair proportion of Dominion and
Colonial troops. Two thousand two hundred
and seven Canadians and more than two thousand
Australian and New Zealand men and about
two hundred U.S.A. troops made up this proportion. They had the same cheerful spirit as
the men in Paris and Wimereux. They settled
down to enjoy the amenities of the hospital with
apparently little thought for the past or the

future, entering into the hospital life with zest
and pleasure ; and their contentment and gaiety
were pleasant to see. Within an hour of coming
in, new-comers learnt that it was ' a good home '
and that the doctors were women. They showed
no surprise, but were wont to develop amazing
confidence in the ward doctors and to discuss
the merits of the various surgeons in the square.
Each man thought his ward the best ward in
the hospital, and his doctor the best doctor on
the staff ; and many boasted to visitors and
at tea-parties that the worst cases in the hospital
were in their ward and under their doctor. The
dental surgeon, whose skill in extraction was
considered marvellous, never failed to thrill the
men, and she was eagerly pointed out to friends
or visitors. The ophthalmic surgeon excited interest too, for she was the victim of a false report,
which supposed her to have broken more windows
than any other suffragist !

Only once did a man ask to be transferred on
the ground that he did not wish to be under a
woman surgeon, but he repented of his decision
and sent his mother to ask that he might remain.
More than once, a transfer was offered in certain
cases, in order that the patient might be treated
by a man ; but this was invariably refused, the

patient feeling perfectly satisfied where he was.
Their confidence in the Chief Surgeon was un-
bounded. She never operated without telling
the patient what she was going to do, and she
never omitted to see him afterwards and talk
over the operation. Between the hours of 5 and
7 P.M. was a quiet and very useful time in the
wards, when she would visit all the more severe
cases and give them time to talk about themselves. She would explain clearly the surgical
situation and what she advised and why. She
never hurried a man in his decision, unless it
were urgent; but waited, gentle and reassuring,
until he would say, ' I leave it to you, Doctor;
if you think it 's best, I 'll have it done.'

The men were reticent and inarticulate, but
they trusted her. They wrote to her afterwards
for advice; and pensioners were known to travel
from Scotland and other distant places to get
her opinion. In the same way, they believed in
and trusted the ward surgeons and the Sisters,
and realised that every one in the building desired
their welfare and happiness. There was a home-
liness in the wards and in the men's relations
with the nursing staff which was soothing and
welcome to them after their experiences.

Racial characteristics were very evident. The

English were slow and phlegmatic, satisfied with theatres, billiards and the football news. The Scots were friends with the librarian and always pushing to get well enough to see London. The Irish brought grace and charm into the ward, but each one was the Irish question intact. Their grievances were as unexpected as they were incomprehensible. As a rule, they were anxious to be transferred to Irish hospitals, and the necessary steps having been taken, Pte. Doolan would receive instructions to draw his kit and prepare himself. Then he would go grumbling up and down the ward.

' But I thought you wanted to go to Ireland,' said an astonished orderly.

' So I do,' he replied. ' But I think this is very hard.' And in response to further probing, ' Well, I did ask to go, but I wasn't expecting to go—not this week.'

Or one would present himself in the C.O.'s office.

' I wish to mak' a complaint. There 's a lot of men in the ward gone to the theatre and the Sister kep' me back.'

Under discussion, it transpired that he was not so well, and being kept in bed, he had risen and dressed to come down and make his complaint.

' It 's true the doctor said I was not to leave my bed, me being with a temperature again.'

When asked whether he would have wished the other men to stay in, since he could not go out, he replied with dignity that he was not ' an onreasonable man ' ; and on being advised to return to his bed and take care of himself, he said :

' Would ye say a wurrrd to the Sister ? '

Then with a ' Thank ye kindly, lady,' he retired to bed again all smiles !

With all their difficulties, they were the most grateful of people. It was the Irish who stood up in the ward and made speeches to the nurses before the Irish convoy left ; and it took an Irishman to say that if he had been all the time in this hospital, he never would have had the heart to leave it, and then to confound the doctor by a bitter complaint at a fancied delay in procuring his transfer.

Australians and New Zealanders began to arrive from Gallipoli in August 1915. They were gaunt and grey after their terrible experiences. The wounded had suffered much during the voyage home, and all of them were wasted with disease. They were big, fine men, reduced by three or more stone below their usual weight, and so weakened by long illness that they lay silent and apathetic in their beds, thankful to be at rest at last. The sick were collected in special wards, and it was not long before they began to put on weight and lift up their heads. The pathologist concentrated on them, and the laboratory had a fine exhibit of lamblia and tetramites and kindred organisms, which excited the interest of the staff. Whenever special diseases were admitted, every one was invited to see the specimens and listen to brief lectures, even the cooks and the librarian's charlady availing themselves of such opportunities !

These men were better educated than the British soldiers. Mentally they were more formed, and were accustomed to independence of thought. Their attitude towards the women, among whom they had been thrown so unexpectedly, was friendly and chivalrous. They enjoyed the hospital and they appreciated the work which was being done there ; but they could not understand why the vote was withheld from women, and in face of their eager questioning the medical staff was unable to adhere completely to its rule of avoiding propaganda talk on the subject of women's suffrage. They were almost the only men who wished to discuss this subject and other political subjects with the doctors and sisters.

As they got better, they were able to go about, and they were greatly interested in London. A party which went to the House of Commons included Pte. King, a keen politician. At the House, various members were introduced to the Australian soldiers, and Mr. Ramsay MacDonald asked the politician what hospital he came from. Hearing that it was Endell Street, he could not resist saying what a great suffragist he was, and how much he had helped the women's cause.

'That may be, sir,' replied Pte. King cautiously, 'but these ladies have records of every M.P.'s career, and they know exactly what each one has done and how he has voted.'

Relating the interview in his ward that night, the politician inquired what this M.P. had done to help; for, he said, 'he seemed properly put about.'

During these weeks, when about two hundred beds were occupied by Australian troops, officers from their headquarters used to call, full of anxiety as to the conduct of their men. The reason of this anxiety was not understood till afterwards, when reports were circulated that there had been difficulty and outbreaks in other hospitals and that Australians were considered 'very wild.' Many Australians were admitted to Endell Street Hospital, but they never gave any trouble. On the contrary, they showed a consideration and courtesy towards the staff which was only equalled by the attitude of the New Zealanders.

Eventually, the hospital became one of those to which New Zealand soldiers were sent, and the wards—especially the medical wards—had many serious cases among them. In the spring of 1917, and again in 1918, a great many cases of pneumonia occurred among New Zealanders, and some of them made marvellous recoveries. These troops were very much liked in the hospital ; for they had gentle, refined manners and a wide outlook, especially where women were concerned. The organisation of the New Zealand Head-quarters was one of the most efficient. It gave no unnecessary trouble to the hospital, and took a great deal of care of its men. In marked con-trast was the Canadian organisation, which dupli-cated and triplicated the work of the offices, and sent innumerable letters of inquiry, instead of filing and referring to hospital returns. With a few exceptions, their men were brusque and somewhat rough, and the medical staff learnt to dislike the manners of Canadian staff officers thoroughly. Among their ranks were men of all nationalities—Russians, Greeks and Japanese, with whom communication was difficult, as they did not know English, and many Frenchmen, who spoke a *patois* only. These latter would have been very friendless, if Monsieur and Madame de Bry had not been available close at hand in their chocolate shop, and a message to them was never sent in vain. On visiting days the French soldiers were sure of seeing either Madame de Bry or one of the charming young ladies who sold so many sweets to the orderlies at Endell Street.

In 1919, when men were evacuated from Russia by Archangel and England, a party of French infantrymen arrived in an ambulance, with a large dog on a very stout rope. He was very gentle with people, but as he had lived in the forest camps and been trained to kill bears, he was not to be trusted with other dogs, and there was a hectic moment in Tottenham Court Road when he met a bull terrier, and two men and the rope were required to hold him. A party of Greeks and another of Serbians also came from Russia, the latter rejoicing in the sights and shops of London.

In that year, too, numbers of cases came from the East and from India, and it was not unusual to meet a monkey or a parrot or a strange reptile harbouring in the wards for a few days.

In August 1917 sixty beds were set aside for women, and were available for Q.M.A.A.C. and other women's units until January 1919. Ladies who had been working abroad with the Y.M.C.A. or canteens found hospitality at Endell Street, and the wives of officers and N.C.O.'s, with children and little babies and their governesses and their nurses, returning from the East, spent a few days there. In all, two thousand women passed through those wards.

Comparatively few Americans were admitted as patients, but in the summer of 1919 orders were sent to accommodate a hundred and fifty U.S.A. troops, not sick, on their way home from Russia. These men, to judge by their names, were mostly of Russian origin. The U.S.A. Headquarters telephoned to the hospital to keep the men in for inspection, but consented to letting them go out the second day. The men were inclined to paint the town red, and straggled back, drunk and sorry, up till 1 A.M. The Headquarters said they must stay in next day, as they might leave at any moment. But no orders for departure came through, and the men became restless and rebellious and would have broken hospital but for the persuasive feminine tongue, which led them back to their wards. They were granted leave to go out the next day and were started off for U.S.A. on the following morning, less half-a-dozen who did not return in time, and two who were in the hands of the police for firing revolvers in the streets.

The critics and the sceptics prophesied that women would fail in keeping discipline, and certainly the War Office did nothing to strengthen their hands. It denied the women commissions or honorary rank, and refused to let them wear the badges of rank which soldiers recognise as symbols of authority. Thus there was nothing except her bearing to distinguish a senior from a junior officer. It would have been helpful if an experienced warrant officer had been appointed to the hospital, but instead a newly promoted corporal was put in charge of the R.A.M.C. detachment. Having thus made it as difficult as possible, the authorities left the women to sink or swim. But discipline came of itself. Until 1919 no conscious effort was made to maintain it, and in that year it only became necessary to take definite trouble about it owing to the very large numbers of men transferred to the hospital from others which were closing and in which a certain laxity had prevailed.

It was very rare for a man to be reported for a small offence and brought before the C.O., and in the early days the embarrassment was mutual. The sergeant (afterwards the sergeant-major) was often asked to leave the offender alone with her, so that she could speak more freely ; and an appeal to the feelings of the sinner generally reduced him to tears. Then he had to be detained in the office with more pleasant conversation, till he regained his composure sufficiently to meet the public eye. After such an interview, one young fellow retired to his bed, and drawing the blankets over his head, refused to answer the inquiries of his much concerned friends. In the evening, when hunger drew him from his lair, they gathered round him with solicitude.

' I 've been up before men and up before women,' he said, ' and God save us from the women ! '

The conduct of the hospital was based upon the Army rules for men in military hospitals ; and now and then, when things were not going quite well in a ward, the N.C.O. patients would be paraded in the office and the Doctor-in-Charge would read to them the rule making N.C.O.'s responsible for ward discipline. With a few

words about the hospital and the staff who cared
so much for its reputation, she would enlist
their interest and help. As they themselves
expressed it, ' After that, there was nothing more
to be done.'

In 1915 to 1916 the Army rule which did not
permit men to go out unconducted was in force,
and walks and drives were extensively organised.
Many friends came several times a week to take
men out, thereby helping to keep them happy
and contented. Foremost among these was
Mrs. Cobden Hirst, who with the help of a
group of hostesses organised hundreds of outings
and gave immense pleasure to several thousand
patients. This rule was subsequently rescinded,
and the order to let men out till 5 P.M., and later
till sundown, was welcomed by all concerned.

It was rare for a man to be late in coming in
or to stay out all night ; for such offences meant
that the privilege of going out would be suspended
for his whole ward next day, and he would have
an uncomfortable time with his fellows. On days
of public rejoicing, such as Armistice Day or
Peace Day, extended privileges were freely given,
but they were not abused. On Peace night
every man was in by 10 P.M. ; not one was absent.
This punctuality was perhaps due to a large tea,

with sausages and tomatoes and cake in the afternoon, and to a meal of cocoa and eggs at 10 P.M. These luxuries having been advertised in the wards the day before, the men knew where comfort was to be found. In any case, things went smoothly. The life of the hospital was not dull. Festivities and Bank Holidays were observed. There was an endless succession of outings — drives, teas and theatres; within, the library was an important interest, the needlework a constant pleasure; and the two or three entertainments given every week were eagerly looked forward to. There was always something going on, or something coming on, which kept the men interested and expectant.

CHAPTER III

MEDICAL AND SURGICAL WORK

FROM the professional point of view, the work which came into the hospital was excellent : it was varied and full of interest, and it gave women an exceptional opportunity in the field of surgery. The responsibility for finding the medical and surgical staff rested with the Doctor-in-Charge, the War Office confirming the appointments on her recommendation. By a special arrangement these appointments were binding for six months at a time, and could then be renewed or terminated as desired. The medical officers were not commissioned, but they were graded as lieutenants, captains, majors or lieut.-colonel, and each one drew the pay and allowances, under Royal Pay Warrant, of her respective rank. They also drew uniform allowance and specialist pay, as well as the bonus and new rates of pay when these were introduced. On the termination of their service they were granted a gratuity.

Among the graduates who served at Endell

Street were representatives of the Universities of England, Scotland, Canada and Australia. Some of them spent one year or two years there. Others continued for the whole period that the hospital was open. The general knowledge which all the doctors were able to have of all the work in the hospital, and especially of all the serious cases, was a great advantage. The ward officers acted as orderly officer in rotation — that is, they took casualties and night work for twenty-four hours in rotation—and had the supervision of the wards on their nights on duty. In civil hospitals members of the staff may not meet for weeks at a time ; but in a military hospital surgeons and physicians attended daily, and at the morning meeting the orderly officer's report for the previous night was read, and it was possible to talk over the various cases. A great deal of good team work was done, the surgeons, physician and pathologist concentrating on the worst cases. The pathological laboratory, which was situated in the centre of the square, was the scene of many useful consultations.

Of the five hundred and seventy-three beds, sixty were reserved for medical cases, and the other five hundred and thirteen were under the supervision of the Chief Surgeon. Each of her assis-

L

tants had charge of sixty or seventy beds, and one ward was generally given to the Doctor-in-Charge, who refused to be excluded altogether from professional work.

The surgeons spent all their mornings in the wards, and most of their afternoons in the operating theatre, where it was not unusual to have a list of twenty or thirty cases on each operating day.

In 1915 large numbers of wounds of head, presenting many interesting features, were admitted. From the surgeon's point of view they were fine cases, for they did well. One lad, who had a bullet removed $1\frac{1}{4}$ inches deep from the brain, was found sitting up sewing at his badge four days afterwards, and greatly pleased with himself.

After steel helmets came into use these injuries decreased in number, and other kinds of wounds took their place. There were always an immense number of compound fractures, for three hundred of the surgical beds were returned as orthopædic. And in 1917 one hundred and fifty-four compound fractured thighs were in the wards at the same time. These were exacting cases: a good result depended on the excellence of the nursing and the most unremitting surgical care

and watchfulness. The latest forms of apparatus
were manufactured by the carpenter, Mr. J. A.
Campbell of Arduaine, and the masseuses toiled
over the patients without ceasing. The results
were very satisfactory, and it was disappointing
to be told, in 1918, that in future fractures of
thigh were to be grouped in special hospitals.
However, that same year brought in a series of
wounds of knee-joint which exercised the ingenuity
and skill of all concerned. In addition, there was
valuable experience with fractures of the upper arm.

The wounded owed much to the inventive genius
of Mrs. Banks. She began work in the hospital
mending room, and then became famous over
papier mâché. No one could construct splints
for the upper arm so comfortably and so effect-
ively as she did, and her abdominal belts and
other appliances were greatly appreciated. One
notable case had the humerus smashed into a
hundred pieces, but it ultimately united and the
patient left hospital with a useful arm and some
X-ray photographs which thrilled him. There
were men with divided or injured nerves, and
several hundreds with acute appendicitis, both
interesting and satisfactory to the surgeon ;
besides all the more ordinary gunshot injuries,
many of them with fractures, for which the

operations of wiring and plating the bones were constantly undertaken.

The number of operations performed in the theatres was seven thousand, but the minor ones done in the wards or casualty room were unrecorded, and are not included in this figure.

When the wards were full of men, the actual work of dressing their wounds occupied a great deal of time ; and as it was often necessary that a large number should be dressed twice a day, or even every four hours, the work was never finished.

In July 1916, at a time when the hospital was very crowded and dressing was going on practically all day, Professor R. Morrison, of Newcastle on Tyne, wrote to the pathologist, asking that his method of using ' Bipp ' might have a trial. Doctors, nurses and patients alike were finding the constant changing of dressings exhausting, and suggestions were welcome. ' Bipp ' was a paste which, after being rubbed into the wound, could be left untouched for ten or even twenty-one days. A chemical reaction kept up an antiseptic effect, and the undisturbed tissues healed rapidly. The first results were so romantic that an extended trial was given to the method ; and before long ' Bipp ' came into general use in the hospital and held its position first amongst all other disinfectants. The work in the wards at once became manageable ; the number of dressings fell 80 per cent, and the results were splendid. The men appreciated the rest and relief from painful dressings and were also proud of their rapid progress. New-comers might look doubtful when they heard that their wounds would be left alone for ten days, and would murmur that in the last hospital they were dressed every day ; but their neighbours had learnt to comment on old-fashioned ways, and laughed them out of their fears. ' Bipp ' metamorphosed the work of the hospital. The surgeons relied on it so confidently that they never hesitated to operate on septic fractures or joints ; and on one occasion a scalp abscess was evacuated, the skull trephined and a bullet extracted from the brain, in the complete assurance that ' Bipp ' would save the situation, as it did.

In the autumn of the year 1916 Sir Alfred Keogh paid his first and only visit to Endell Street. He came, accompanied by the Deputy Director of Medical Services for the London District, to see the results obtained by the use of ' Bipp ' ; for the War Office had heard of the method and was considering introducing it into the Army hospitals and casualty clearing stations abroad. Endell Street was the only hospital in London which had given it an extensive trial, and it was a proud moment when the Chief Surgeon led the Director General from ward to ward, displaying one good surgical result after another, showing normal temperature charts and healed wounds, with conservation of tissues and good movements. At last he said that he had seen enough and was convinced, and when he took his leave, he congratulated the staff upon the success of the hospital.

'I knew you could do it,' he said. 'We were watched, but you have silenced all critics.'

In his busy life, Sir Alfred Keogh had not time to see the hospital again, but he kept himself informed of its progress, and when the time came that he left the War Office, he wrote as follows :

DEAR DR. GARRETT ANDERSON—I appreciate very highly the very charming message you and Doctor Flora Murray have sent me in your letter. I shall go down to see you and say good-bye before I actually leave the War Office.

I should have liked to have seen you and your work very often, but you will know that with six foreign campaigns on hand, and an immense amount of work in addition in connection with home affairs—which perhaps were even more difficult than the foreign ones—it has not been possible for me to visit you more than I have done. I have not been unmindful of you I can assure you. I have often talked of you and heard your work discussed, and it has always been to me a great pride to know how successful you have been.

I was subjected to great pressure adverse to your movement when we started to establish your Hospital, but I had every confidence that the new idea would justify itself, as it has abundantly done. Let me, therefore, thank you and Doctor Flora Murray—not only for what you have done for the country, but for what you have done for me personally. I should have been an object of scorn and ridicule if you had failed, but I never for a moment contemplated failure, and I think we can now congratulate ourselves on having established a record of a new kind.

I think your success has probably done more for the cause of women than anything else I know of, and if that cause flourishes, you and I can feel that we have been sufficiently rewarded for our courage.—Yours sincerely,

ALFRED KEOGH.

19th January 1918.

It was characteristic of the Women's Hospital Corps that, when the Director General had left the hospital—or, indeed, after any official visitor had left—various members of the staff would come to the office, one after the other, to ask how the inspection had gone, and to rejoice over any little word of praise or appreciation which might have been given to their hospital.

About three weeks after the hospital opened two severe cases of acute mania were admitted. As there was no ground-floor ward and no window with any protection, they were a source of anxiety to the medical staff. One of them was blasphemous and homicidal, the other deeply religious and suicidal ; both were violent and noisy and had to be detained in a small room by themselves, with several R.A.M.C. men in constant attendance. The hospital telephoned to the Horse Guards, reporting the matter and asking instructions as to their disposal, and was told that instructions would be sent. The next day the hospital telephoned again for instructions, and the reply was that the men must not be certified. On the third day the hospital telephoned urgently and inquired about disposal. It was told that the question was under consideration and that information would be sent. On the fourth day the hospital telephoned still more urgently and received the same reply. It telephoned again the same afternoon, and this time was told that Colonel H—— would come and see the Doctor-in-Charge.

Towards five o'clock, a gentle and very elderly colonel arrived. Evidently, he was under the impression that women doctors were unaccustomed to lunatics and were unduly alarmed.

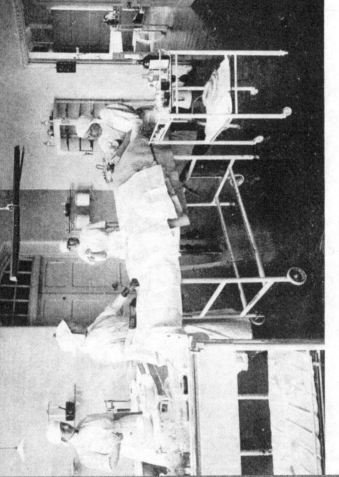

IN THE OPERATING THEATRE

(Page 170)

(Photo, Reginald Haines)

AN INSPECTION IN THE DENTAL ROOM

(Photo, Reginald Haines)

(Page 171)

'Yes, mental cases,' he said, 'rather worry you, don't they ? Yes, yes, not nice cases for ladies. I will just go up and say a soothing word to them—poor fellows.'

The Doctor-in-Charge and Chief Surgeon looked at each other and then led the colonel upstairs.

Pte. T—— was sitting up in bed, cadaverous and morose, and behind the screen the orderlies were struggling to prevent Pte. W—— from choking himself while he recited his prayers. The colonel spoke soothingly to Pte. T——, but obtained no response. Pte. T—— only continued to glare fiercely. So he passed round the screen to see Pte. W——. Immediately, Pte. T——, stealthily and rapidly, got out of bed, and prowling after the colonel, seized him from behind ! The orderlies interfered and a regular scrimmage ensued, until the doctors, who were almost helpless with laughter, seeing that the officer was being roughly used, called in further help, and a dishevelled, flustered colonel was assisted out of the room.

'Dear me, they are indeed dangerous fellows,' he said. 'We had no idea they were so bad.'

He went straight back to the Horse Guards. And very promptly orders were sent for the removal of the patients to safer quarters without delay.

The work in the medical wards was perhaps less dramatic than on the surgical side, but it was not less severe. Many cases of rheumatism, gastric ulcer and cardiac disease spent weeks in the hospital, and pleurisy and empyema were constantly admitted. There were painful cases of gas poisoning and malaria, and others of mental disturbance; but pneumonia dominated the wards in numbers and in severity. They were anxious cases, occurring constantly among New Zealand and Australian men, whose distance from their homes made a further claim on the sympathies of the staff. Recovery depended largely upon the nursing, and many of them owed their lives to the devoted work of Sister Hughes and Sister Exell, who were in charge of St. Felicitas and St. Geneviève wards.

During the first two years the physician in charge of the medical side was Dr. Louisa Woodcock. When she died in February 1917, the staff lost one of its most brilliant and successful members. She was a woman of high professional attainment, of scientific mind and of noble character. Her influence in the hospital was always helpful, and her friendship was greatly valued and greatly missed by her colleagues. She was succeeded by Dr. Margaret Thackrah, who was appointed in May, and when the number of medical beds was increased in 1919, Dr. Ellen Pickard also joined the staff.

The women's wards, at the top of the East Block, were the best in the hospital, and as the women were less destructive than men, it was easy to make them homelike and comfortable. The arrangement to take women was initiated as a temporary measure, but it continued for more than two years. The work was both surgical and medical. The recruiting for the women's units had not always been prudent, and many women were sent home unfit, as the result of illnesses or operations occurring before enlistment. Most of these came before Invaliding Boards and were discharged. But the greater number of the patients sent home from France were debilitated, or anæmic and fatigued by long hours and an unaccustomed diet, and needed rest and good conditions to make them ready for service again. A rather large proportion of mental cases, all of whom had had previous attacks, and some serious injuries owing to accidents and to the bombing of camps, were received. The women's wards were the most responsive wards in the hospital. They were credulous of rumours and false reports, suscept-

ible to the influence of a 'grouser' or a change
of Sister, but on the other hand they responded
readily to wise handling, and were led and guided
by their ward visitor, Mrs. Prior.

During the influenza epidemics of 1918 and 1919
men and women suffering from the disease trooped
into the casualty room or sent messages for ambulances to fetch them. The extra beds were all
full, and the number of men seriously ill with
pneumonia might be fifty or sixty each day.
The staff slaved over them. Extra nurses were
procured; the doctors knew no rest. But the
mortality was tremendous. In the months of
November and December 1918 twenty-four men
and women died; and in February 1919 thirty
died. The hospital was accustomed to a death
rate of eight per thousand per annum, and was
aghast over three deaths in one day. Sorrowing
and anxious relatives sat in the square and passages, watching the doctors' faces as they went
in and out of the wards, and patiently accepting
the issue. Old people who had never been out
of Ireland came over, and would not venture in
the streets in case they should be lost or run over.
Grey - haired fathers and mothers came from
Scotland to sit, silent and enduring, beside the
beds. The habitual gaiety of the place was hidden

under the cloud. The staff could only work and wait. A dear old uncle and aunt arrived from the country to see a precious nephew, whose life hung in the balance for some days. One morning the doctor met them in the square and told them that their boy was better and should do well now. They both burst into tears, and presently the old lady, through her sobs, begged the doctor to excuse 'Uncle,' for 'he was always so silly and took on so.'

Pte. B——, a Scottish shepherd, had wounds of hip and knee, and was so ill that his wife was sent for. She travelled all night, and for twenty-four hours sat steadily beside his bed. When it was suggested to her that she was tired and should lie down, Pte. B—— opened his eyes to say, ' Och ! the wife's enjoying herself fine, sitting beside me here.'

The relatives were very brave and very pathetic. The men clung to their mothers, and many a careworn, weary woman sat night after night by the side of her son, grateful because she was allowed to be there.

The hospital had its share of malingerers and self-inflicted injuries, and one or two cases of fraud. The cleverest of these was a man admitted for some slight ailment, who had only one arm, and who stated that he was awaiting admission to a limbless hospital. He was in the ward for ten days, and might have left undetected but for the thoroughness of the Chief Surgeon, who insisted upon seeing whether the stump was in a good condition before he left. The Sister said he was a very modest man and did not like to show his arm to ladies.

'Surely he need not be modest about an arm,' said the Surgeon. And the Sister unfastened his jacket.

'Which arm did you say, Sister?' she continued. 'He seems to have the usual number.'

And so he had. He stood abashed before a half-fainting Sister, while Dr. Garrett Anderson and the orderlies pealed with laughter, and the whole ward joined in the joke.

The amount of clerical work required of the doctors was no light matter. They had to keep all the notes for their own beds, and as the turn-over was generally fairly rapid, the writing was incessant. Convalescent men reported to the office of the Doctor-in-Charge for discharge on two days a week, and history sheets had to be made up for every one who left or was transferred.

The monthly turn-over varied between four hundred and eight hundred cases, and each admission and each discharge or transfer entailed the preparation and despatch of several forms. Invaliding Boards were held regularly, and thirty-nine different forms had to be filled up and signed for each man who came before the Board. As time went on, the work of these Boards became heavier ; for the Army Council was clever at inventing new forms. But when once the Ministry of Pensions got into its stride, these were triplicated and amplified, and the hospital's responsibilities in clothing, equipping and providing for the men were largely increased.

The War Office had a habit of issuing numbers of circular instructions to hospitals, many of which dealt with medical subjects. These were known at Endell Street as ' purple papers,' from the colour of their ink, and it was usual to post them in the Staff Room, where they sometimes gave rise to amusement. One circular warned surgeons against using syringes without sterilising them first, and suggested that for this purpose ' a little warm oil ' should be used ; another pointed out that they should not make a practice of amputating the right arm, unless it were absolutely necessary to do so ; while a third informed them that ' death under an anæsthetic ' should in future be regarded as part of the treatment.

The Army has a wonderful way of having an official name and number for each disease. These are to be found in the official ' Nomenclature of Diseases,' and no patient may have any disease not mentioned in the book. For instance, the Army does not recognise rheumatism, and many soldiers had to have ' 37 Rheumatic Fever ' or ' 931 Myalgia ' instead. On the other hand, the book had some nice comprehensive diagnoses, such as ' 952 I.C.T. (inflammation of connective tissue) ' and ' 21 P.U.O. (Pyrexia of uncertain origin),' which were very useful in haste. The proper nomenclature and numbers were much insisted upon by the Medical Statistical Department, and tired doctors sometimes felt that the extra work which had to be done for this department was almost the last straw.

Three auxiliary V.A.D. hospitals—at Dollis Hill, under the Commandant, Mrs. Richardson, O.B.E., and at Highgate, under the Commandant, Lady Crosfield, R.R.C.—were a great source of pleasure and benefit to the men. When fully expanded, these hospitals provided, under fine conditions, a hundred and fifty beds for the more conval-

escent cases. They were very popular with the
men, who were well cared for and very happy in
them ; and as an important factor in recovery
they were greatly appreciated by the medical
staff.

M

CHAPTER IV

THE VISITORS—THE ENTERTAINMENTS—
THE LIBRARY

THE Deputy Director of Medical Services for the
London District was the official head of the
hospital, and Endell Street knew three officers
in succession in that capacity. The first of these
was remarkable for his length of limb and the
brevity of his tongue. His frigid attitude might
have been misunderstood at the preliminary
interview, if he had not been accepted as 'very
Scotch' and 'obviously East Coast.' On his
rare visits to the hospital he would stride silently
through the wards, making his round, without
saying more than 'Uch ha!' and a curt 'Good
morning' on leaving. Time led to a slightly
better acquaintance, and on one occasion he
even made a joke about misappropriation, and the
wintry smile that crossed his face was like a gleam
of sunshine in February. His efficiency was
liked, and his habit of returning applications
(although generally marked 'inadmissible') was
very convenient. His successors were less tall

and had more to say, and relations with them were easy and pleasant.

Visitors were nearly as numerous in London as they had been in Paris. The King and Queen honoured the hospital with a visit, and went through the wards giving great pleasure to the patients. More often, Queen Alexandra and Princess Victoria would arrive, either to see the men or to be present at some entertainment. And it was on one of these occasions that an Irishman begged to be allowed to go down to the recreation room.

' For,' said he, ' the only member of the Royal Family that I have seen is Sir Edward Carson, and I would like to see the Queen.'

When Her Majesty heard this, she asked to be taken to his bedside, so that she might speak to him. She was full of kindness and sympathy for the sick, and would give them little books, or smelling-salts from her own reticule, and once she handed her handkerchief to a dying man with which to wipe his face. This handkerchief he gave to his sister, who preserves it as one of the great treasures of Lancashire. After her visits, Queen Alexandra would send gifts for distribution to the men. Among these valued mementos were ash walking-sticks, with silver bands en-

graved with ' A.' One severely wounded man
was found awake at night with his ' Queen's
stick ' in his bed. He had refused the morphia
which had been ordered for him, as he was afraid
to go to sleep lest some one should take his stick.
It was only when safe custody had been promised
for the stick that he consented to rest.

The Princess Royal, the Duke of Connaught
and Princess Arthur of Connaught also came
to the hospital, and Lord French paid a visit
one afternoon, and had many things to say to
the patients.

More frequent and very welcome visitors were
Lieut.-General Sir Francis Lloyd, G.C.V.O., K.C.B.,
D.S.O., and Lady Lloyd. The men enjoyed
seeing them, especially when the General Officer
Commanding made speeches, and the staff of
the hospital much appreciated his kindness and
courtesy. His successor, Major - General Sir
Geoffrey Fielding, K.C.B., C.M.G., D.S.O., and
Lieut.-General Sir T. H. Goodwin, K.C.B., C.M.G.,
D.S.O., who succeeded Sir Alfred Keogh as
Director General, were also among those who
inspected the hospital.

The news that the Chief Magistrate, Sir John
Dickinson, had called, and would return next
day, was disturbing, for relations between magis-
trates and suffragists had not always run

smoothly. The Doctor-in-Charge questioned the quartermaster : ' What do you think the Chief Magistrate can be coming about ? '

' I don't know,' she answered, ' unless it is about that kitchen-maid.' And she told how one of the kitchen staff had been to a dance in her brother's uniform, and, coming home through the streets, had been warned by a policeman.

With this crime on their consciences Sir John's visit was awaited uneasily. But he came in friendship, with outstretched hand and kind congratulations upon the womanly work which his former acquaintances had found to do.

With Endell Street before it as a demonstration, the War Office could not fail to perceive that ward duties and the general administrative work of hospitals came easily within the scope of women. Towards the end of 1915 instructions were circulated to officers in charge of hospitals, requiring them to set free men so employed and to replace them with women. Those in command of military and of naval hospitals began to arrive at the women's hospital, anxious to learn how this might be done. They were given opportunities of seeing women stretcher-bearing, handling bags of sugar and potatoes, or doing fire-drill. Armed with notebooks and pencils, they would make notes of all they saw and sadly discuss what they used to describe as 'the hopeless difficulty of the situation.'

During 1916 and 1917 one staff officer called periodically to see whether every possible man had been replaced by a woman. His time was spent in inspecting hospitals and trying to persuade those in authority to replace their men; and naturally Endell Street was his example. Again and again he came to say that he was assured that it was impossible to use women for certain services, and to ask how it was done. Amongst other things, he had been told that to use women in the X-ray room was 'indelicate.' The Doctor-in-Charge reminded him that skiagrams were made through clothing and in a dark room.

'I never thought of telling them that,' he said.

Talking over his experiences elsewhere, he remarked: 'As soon as I say, "But at Endell Street——" I see a nauseated expression come over their faces.' And his tales of the obstruction he met with among old-fashioned officers and N.C.O.'s were amusing.

Acting on these general orders, the Doctor-in-Charge applied in September 1916 for authority to replace fourteen men by fourteen women. Referring to the R.A.M.C. personnel, she wrote:

The greater number of these men (nineteen) are physically unfit. Their physique is very poor and their work is not satisfactory. I find that able-bodied women are capable of performing practically all the duties which these men perform.

In March 1917 a return showed that three women had replaced four men as dining-hall attendants, one woman had replaced one sergeant as cook, and fourteen women had replaced fourteen men on general duties. Later, the Doctor-in-Charge stated that 'no additional women can be employed in substitution for men in this hospital.' The staff of men had been reduced to two N.C.O.'s and six men, and fourteen young women had been attached to the R.A.M.C. detachment to act under the orders of the sergeant-major.

There was no difficulty about the arrangement. The girls were splendid. They emptied the ward bins, managed the incinerator, removed soiled linen and took up the clean, distributed the dinner wagons, swept and hosed the square, carried stretchers, conducted patients to the stations or travelled with them to Brighton and other places, as required. They rose at night when the convoy bell rang or air-raid warnings came through ; they manned the fire hose and took their turn of night duty and gate duty, with marked efficiency. The sergeant-major praised them highly ; for they were sober, disciplined and industrious. The men and women paraded together, but messed separately ; and the mixed company, which had at first been tried as an experiment, was one of the great successes.

Experience in France had shown that though visitors in the wards were a great help and pleasure, the number and the kind of visitor might easily be harmful, and a decision was taken to regulate the visiting, so as to reserve certain days and hours when quietness might prevail in the wards and when the nurses might be able to give extra care and attention to those who needed it. These regulations were found to be fully justified ; for the many very sick men constantly distributed through the hospital would have suffered more than was right if unlimited visiting had been allowed. In order that there might be dependable visitors, a lady was appointed as official ward visitor to each ward. She became an honorary member of the corps and devoted herself to the interests and welfare of the men in her ward.

'I want to ask you a question,' said a rather dour sort of man to his ward visitor when she came to his bedside.

' Yes, what is it ? ' she asked, sitting down beside him.

' I want to know what you come for. You come and sit by my bed and talk, and you never talk about religion nor about politics. Now, what do you do it for ? '

When she explained that she did it in the hope of giving him a little change and pleasure, he said : ' Well, I say that it 's wonderful.'

Men confined to bed for long periods looked forward to their visitor's days, and missed them when they were out of town. And many still write to the ladies who gave so much time to this work and who had such a sympathetic understanding of their needs.

The hospital was overwhelmed by visitors of all sorts and conditions, who came at all hours for any purpose and who were all determined to ' speak one word of kindness to the poor fellows,' or, as one lady wrote, ' to bring one ray of pleasure into the lives of the poor mutilated darlings.' There were scores of people representing regimental associations and other societies, who were sure that no one except themselves would say ' a kind word ' or convey ' a little brightness ' into the wards. All of them expected and demanded nominal rolls of men in hospital from the overworked clerks, and they did not

accept it amiably if the 'one man they wanted
to see' was out. It was difficult to make people
realise that wards must close at 5 P.M., since there
were nursing and dressing to do.

'Oh, I am not at all upset by painful sights,'
they would say.

And it was still more difficult to make them
understand that the men could not be disturbed
late in the evening. Officers, Members of Parliament, countesses, ladies who claimed to have
been 'born and bred in the Army,' ladies with
husbands 'in the Blues' or the War Office,
colonels' wives and V.A.D. commandants, were
apt to arrive at 8 P.M. or even later, expecting to
be admitted. All these people had to be seen
and dealt with—reasoned with, cajoled and
smoothed down, or otherwise they did not hesitate
to write and worry the War Office about their
grievances. The staff stood as buffers between
the helpless and sick men and those who did not
understand ; and the buffer gets most of the jar.

Impartial witnesses have marvelled at the
patience and self-control of the girls in charge
of the gate. Their post was difficult and onerous.
They were constantly receiving parcels, answering
inquiries, taking telephone calls or running
messages, obtaining reports for relatives, bringing walking cases down at odd hours to see odd

callers in the square, admitting, directing, checking ; they had to convince callers that the man they wanted to see was not in this hospital, or that it was true that another whom they were seeking had been discharged. But most difficult of all tasks was that of tracing men on quite insufficient data.

'I have come to see my father's footman,' said one lady.

'Yes, what is his name?' asked the gate-keeper.

'David.'

'Is that his surname?'

'I don't know. We always called him David.'

'What is his regiment?'

'Oh! a Highland regiment.'

'We have some Black Watch men in. Do you think he is in that?'

'Yes, I think he is perhaps.'

And somehow they found him for her.

The patients' friends came on three days a week, and on fine summer afternoons, when many men were out in the square, there was often an orchestra playing, and fruit and ices were on sale at the canteen in the corner. The blue suits and red or blue umbrellas suspended over those in bed gave an air of gaiety to the scene which had an almost continental aspect.

Amusements were regarded as of special importance, and Miss Bessie Hatton was asked to be the Honorary Organiser and Secretary of this department, a post which she held until the hospital closed. The hospital was fortunate in securing her help, for she was in touch with the theatrical world, and her delightful gifts as a writer of charming little plays and as an actress of exceptional power made her advice and her experience invaluable. She formed a committee of experts, which was joined by Dame May Whitty, Miss Lilian Braithwaite, Miss Inez Bensusan, Miss Waldegrave and Mrs. J. T. Grein. The latter wrote plays and pantomimes for the hospital and took infinite pains over rehearsals and over the training of a ' troupe ' of gifted girls, whose performances as the ' Endell Street Follies ' were immensely popular. This committee was responsible for the entertainments and music on the stage and in the wards, for Christmas festivities and Bank holiday parties, and for the organisation of the ' Endell Street Orchestra ' under its conductor, Mrs. Salaman.

On summer evenings crowds assembled in the square to listen to the band playing. The patients were equally appreciative of the beautiful singing of the Temple Church choir, of conjurers, reciters or Miss Italia Conti's pretty dancing

children. And performances held in the open-
air had the added advantage that every one in
the wards could hear and enjoy the music and
singing, and that the whole hospital participated
in the pleasure.

St. George's Day, St. Patrick's Day, St. Andrew's
Day and Hallowe'en were all celebrated with
special and appropriate features.

On Bank holidays the patients invited their own
friends to come to tea and spend the afternoon,
and a variety entertainment was arranged to promote the holiday feeling. At Christmas there
were concerts and variety shows, and Mrs. Grein's
pantomime delighted all beholders. Mystery
plays and masques, whist-drives, sports and many
other kinds of fun were introduced and eagerly
taken up.

' I never knew,' said one, ' that it was possible
to have such pleasure and enjoy ourselves so
much without being drunk ! '

A beautiful pageant was arranged in 1915,
representing the Patron Saints of the wards.
Miss Waldegrave as St. Mary led the procession,
and each saint entered preceded by her banner-
bearer. St. Barbara, the patron saint of Arms,
and St. Felicitas with her seven sons, were followed by the Abbess Hildegarde and St. Joan
of Arc. Rachel, surrounded by an international

group of children, and St. Ursula with her band
of noble maidens completed a very interesting
and artistic spectacle.

The recreation room was a moving sight when
it was packed to its uttermost by an eager and
happy audience. On one side of the gangway
were men in beds, and ranks of wheel-chairs with
their more convalescent occupants ; on the other,
a solid mass of men in blue were crowded on chairs,
window-sills or tables, wherever a corner could
be found ; and at the back, a few members of
the staff found standing room. The audience
listened with rapt attention to the singing of
Mr. Courtice Pounds, Miss Jean Sterling Mac-
Kinlay and Miss Grainger Kerr ; or followed the
performances of Sir Johnston Forbes-Robertson,
Mr. H. B. Irving, Miss Ellis Jeffreys, Mr. Nigel
Playfair and Miss Helen Haye with great delight.
The laughter and cheers which greeted each
item marked their appreciation and pleasure.
The programmes were never long, so that patients
who were less well could be included in the fun,
and many of them tried to get better in time
for the entertainments. More than a thousand
artistes visited the hospital each year, and between May 1915 and May 1919 five hundred
and eleven entertainments were held. During
these years the Committee arranged two hundred

and sixty concerts; seventy ward concerts; ninety - five orchestras; fifty - two plays; four pantomimes; and thirty sing-songs.

The King and Queen gave a party to wounded soldiers at Buckingham Palace, to which a number of Endell Street patients were invited. There was a sumptuous tea, followed by a wonderful variety entertainment—an all-star show. of the very best. When the men returned, having thoroughly enjoyed themselves, one of them admitted :

'Yes, they did us very well; but of course we had seen all the turns before on our own stage.'

The hospital owed a great deal to the many artistes who so generously came again and again to amuse and interest the patients.

In the wards reserved for serious cases there were always men whose beds could not be moved to the recreation room, and these found pleasure and amusement through the electrophone installed beside their beds. Every evening men who were still suffering greatly forgot their pain for a time as they lay with the receivers fastened over their ears, listening to 'The Bing Boys' or other plays. It was delightful to see them laughing, and often they fell asleep and were unaware of the night-nurse when she came round and removed the apparatus from their heads. New-comers were always eager to share in this treat, and a man who had just arrived and was having an operation done in the afternoon made his neighbours in the ward promise to rouse him when the time came for 'The Bing Boys.' His surgeon, visiting the ward in the evening, was surprised to find him propped up in bed, with a smile on his face and the receiver on his head.

But daily occupations and interests had to be provided for those who were confined to the hospital for long periods, and to supply this want basket-weaving, knitting, rug-making and needle-work were introduced. Lady Anderson and a small committee of ladies organised the needle-work and found that the embroidery done by the men was quite unexpectedly good. About seven thousand regimental badges were worked, but those who had any aptitude were not re-stricted to this kind of sewing only. Miss Rosa-mond S. Wigram produced designs copied from old pieces of needlework or from pictures, and taught the men how to do needlework pictures. Some who had never sewed before developed great skill, and worked baskets of flowers in excellent shading, or gardens full of colour, and having learnt to make French knots, they

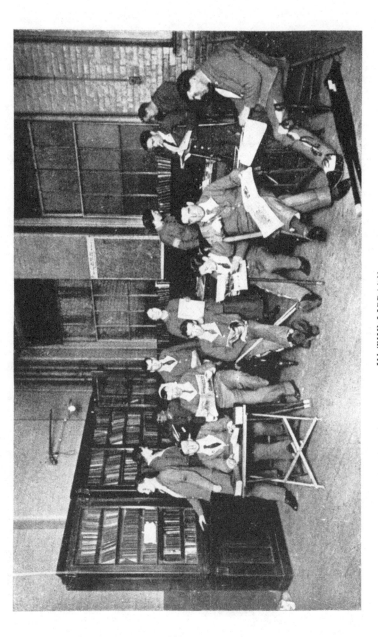

IN THE LIBRARY

(Photo, *Topical Press*)

(Page 196)

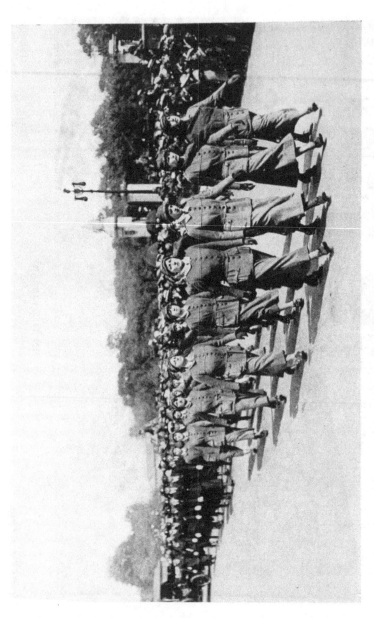

ORDERLIES IN PROCESSION GOING TO BUCKINGHAM PALACE

(Page 197)

(Photo, Central News)

produced life-like woolly lambs and rabbits. The
workers became happily absorbed in their work,
and would take up their sewing frames as soon
as it was light and only lay them aside when it
grew dark. Each year a sale of the work done
for the committee was held, at which some of
the pictures fetched a price of five and seven
guineas each.

Before the Endell Street Hospital opened in
1915, Miss Beatrice Harraden and Miss Elizabeth
Robins were requested to join the staff as Honorary librarians, and the value of the library which
they created cannot be over-estimated. The
important educative influence which it exercised
was due to the personal work of Miss Beatrice
Harraden, who spent many hours daily among
the men, sacrificing, during the whole period
of the hospital's existence, her own work and her
leisure to their needs. Miss Robins was unfortunately unable to continue her help for
long, but in the first weeks Miss Harraden and
she made a fine collection of books and organised
an ambulatory service for the wards. Magazines,
newspapers, stationery, stamps, and very often
matches, were supplied freely by the librarian,
and the demands made upon this department
were so heavy that it was necessary to give

N

Miss Harraden two assistants, and in addition she was glad of the help which Miss Evelyn Glover gave in the afternoons.

At all hours of the day the librarians were to be met in the wards, getting orders for books, and giving advice or encouragement. Miss Harraden used to talk to the men till they felt that they wanted to read the books she spoke of. She catered for every taste : the old reader and the new reader were equally stimulated. Beginning with *Tit Bits* or *Blighty*, by way of Charles Garvice and W. W. Jacobs, they were led along the path of literature till they found themselves absorbed in *Henry VIII.* or Bacon's *Essays* !

A proportion of the patients were educated men, with literary tastes, to whom a good library made all the difference. Six subscriptions at Mudie's were taken out and placed at the disposal of such readers ; so that books could be changed daily if necessary. The rule of the library was to provide every book asked for, on whatever subject and in whatever language. If these books were not in the library or obtainable at Mudie's, Miss Harraden knew where to find them, and many valuable books, on seventeenth-century furniture, old silver, zoology and metaphysics, were lent to the hospital. The technical bookcase was well stocked, and those who had trades or hobbies were encouraged to read their own subject. There were many gardeners in the wards, who pored over books on rose - growing, ferns or chrysanthemums, and furious debates would rage as to the relative superiority of their favourite flowers.

Handbooks about motors, aeroplanes and engines were popular, and some men found interest in fossils and archæology. Men who had been in India said that they learnt more about that country from an illustrated book than from living there for seven years, and it was found that there was quite a vogue for the History of Mexico, Dante and *Don Quixote*. Abridged representations of Shakespeare's plays in the recreation room would send up the demand for this author. One or two men studied for the London Matriculation examination whilst in hospital, the librarian finding the text-books and directing their course. To most of them, reading proved a great source of interest and a great education. Some, it is true, appraised the value of literature by its price ! One man, who had been devoted to reading tales published at twopence and had been persuaded to read one of

H. Seton Merriman's books in the sevenpenny edition, told the librarian that 'this sevenpenny author is an improvement on the twopenny ones. Perhaps I might try something better now. Have you a shilling author I could have ? '

'Oh! why did they bring me back ? Why didn't they let me die ? ' groaned a poor young fellow, restlessly moving his head on his pillow. The presence of the librarian by his bed roused his interest. He was a musician, and he asked her to bring him the life of a musician. She brought *The Life of Chopin*, and a smile came over his face as she placed it in his hands. That afternoon, still smiling and still holding the book between his hands, he passed peacefully away.

In a neighbouring ward a man described himself as a sociologist, and said that the subject he wished to read was 'one which you will not know anything about here.' It was Woman's Suffrage ! With all her years of suffrage work behind her, Miss Harraden said nothing, but produced the books required. A few days later, she asked him : 'Why did you think that we knew nothing about Woman's Suffrage here ? ' and went on to tell him something of the practical interest which she herself and other members of the hospital staff took in that movement.

'But none of you ever talk about it,' the man exclaimed with astonishment. And he listened earnestly while she showed him how the propaganda was going on all the time, though it was a propaganda of deeds and not of words.

The book-cases were not locked, and men could handle the books and choose for themselves, and the staff also had free access at all times and made great use of the privilege. Some books were lost; but the main object of the library was to promote reading, and the losses were accepted quietly. There were generally five thousand books in the library and large surplus stocks were sent away periodically to start libraries in other hospitals and to supplement those in Y.W.C.A. huts and munition factories. The librarian brought real education to the bedside, and aroused intelligence and interest in a wonderful degree.

CHAPTER V

THE WOMEN ORDERLIES

THE mention of the staff of the hospital calls up a picture of that splendid band of young women who responded to the call of patriotism and who, laying aside their habits of ease and pleasure, gave themselves up to the strenuous toil and restricted life of those who serve in hospitals. It is true that the staff included doctors, matron, and trained nurses ; but they were professional people, carrying out their professional work ; and though each and all of them took her share and played her part well, their effort did not compare with that of the young girls, who took up the burden as a simple duty.

The women orderlies who served in the various departments gave the hospital its distinctive character and were largely responsible for the fine spirit which kept all ranks united in such complete harmony and good-fellowship. They were young, and they brought the grace and charm of youth inside the grey walls. Some of them were beautiful and all of them looked charming in their uniform, with their fine physique, their shining hair and look of freedom and self-determination. Their attitude recalled the words of the poet :

> She had the step of the unconquered, brave,
> Not arrogant ; and if the vessel's mast
> Waved liberty, no challenge did it wave.

Gently nurtured, expensively but ineffectively educated, they were unequipped and untrained ; but they had fine courage, and did not lack resolution and intelligence, and, with a little training, they took responsibility in the wards and tackled any difficulty or any situation on the administrative side. They brought laughter into the wards. Their very aspect was cheering. They encouraged, protected, chaffed, and sympathised. Their gaiety was infectious, and their willingness a thing that could be counted on.

The men felt their influence ; but it was only the Australians who could put their feelings into words.

'Disciplined women,' said Sergt. Peto. 'I have never seen such women. Ours can't touch them.'

And it was not only their beauty and their kindness that counted, for they worked hard and well. They controlled the wards in the absence of the Sister ; they managed the sick or wilful, and they were dignified or motherly, authoritative or persuasive, at need. The wounded depended upon them and trusted them, and in return, sought for complimentary interpretations of the ' W.H.C.' on their shoulder-straps. The ' What-Ho-Corps,' ' Wounded Heroes' Comforters,' and suchlike, were meant appreciatively.

At the gate, in the stores, in the offices, they had one desire and one intention—to make the hospital a success. They worked early and late, at dull, ever-repeating tasks, in inconvenient quarters, with humour and with laughter. And out of hours, the residential parts of the building resounded with merriment. They slept, and rose again with shouts of talk and laughter, reassuring to those who feared that the hard work might be too much for them.

The main office was a centre of life, where a cheerful clamour of voices would arise, regardless of open doors ; and tales would be told by one and another of how the Doctor-in-Charge had looked or spoken in different circumstances, and how awful it was, and how funny. They rocked with mirth and capped the stories, till at last a voice from the other office across the passage broke in : ' I am sure I didn't say it like that.'

Then a sudden silence fell, followed by subdued laughter. And one by one grey figures flitted right and left, and business was resumed. To the end of the time, those girls never remembered the open door nor the Doctor-in-Charge working in the adjacent office !

In the quartermaster's offices there was a young team, full of good spirits and ready for any enterprise. They fed and clothed and administered the hospital, and were ready for every entertainment and piece of fun. They prepared extra teas and extra suppers ; rehearsed and performed, if need be ; danced or sang, or carried tables and handed refreshments, with equal vigour and enthusiasm. Messages of appreciation came to the stores from the wards : letters of thanks for special teas, requests for tomatoes or other dainties. Or a sergeant would come to the clothing store, to say that the men in his ward were obliged for being clothed so quickly, and especially for the trouble taken to give them the proper sizes. Men who had left would write with confidence to the quartermaster for jerseys, socks, cakes, musical instruments, belts and other wants, and in answer she constantly sent parcels to France and Salonika.

It was the orderlies who made the special atmosphere of the hospital and who kept its standard of conduct high. Though young in years, they were wonderfully sensible. Their duties were performed with friendliness and charm, but with unfailing dignity, and no man ever took liberties or caused them inconvenience.

They threw themselves readily into amusements for the wards, and under their guidance, men dressed up and played parts, while others sang and recited. Sports and games were organised, and the designs for Christmas decorations owed much to their suggestions and ingenuity.

They formed a choir which sang carols in the square at Christmas time, and which on Christmas Eve clothed itself in white dominoes and hoods, and bearing gaily coloured lanterns, passed singing from ward to ward. This little procession of white-robed girls singing the familiar old carols in their sweet voices touched many of the men. One of them told his nurse next day that when it had passed he had said his prayers, ' though he didn't usually.'

An Australian described his arrival at the hospital, when he was on leave in London and felt unwell.

' When I went in at the gate, a flapper asked me what I had come for. Then she called another flapper to take me to the sick-room. I found another flapper there, and she took my temperature and told me to sit down. Then she brought another flapper, and she said I should go into a ward. So I was taken upstairs, and there were more of them. And I 'm blest ! if another flapper didn't come and stand by my bed and write my medicine down.'

But he stayed long enough to become much attached to the ' flapper's hospital.'

' What beats me,' he said, ' is that they all go on as though they had been doing it always.'

This was true ; for each one learnt her part or her office very quickly, and carried on her work with a sense of responsibility and without self-consciousness.

The orderlies showed a great power of endurance. Many of them remained at work for four and a half years, while others stayed for three or two years. It was rare to have any one leave under one and a half years. Miss Anderson, Miss Nicholson, and Miss Paul nursed right through. They were among the first to come and the last to go. Miss Chance and Miss Tanner gave four years, many months of which were spent in the operating theatre. Miss Joyce Ward joined up at the beginning, aged sixteen, as a messenger, and finished in November 1919, as head financial clerk. There were many others who did equally well, and more than one girl asked to have a vacancy reserved for her before her last term at school was ended. There were failures, but they were allowed to go and were forgotten. There were disappointments, but they were grieved over in silence. The bulk of the girls inspired pride and admiration in those who looked on.

The management disliked rules, and none were drafted for the guidance of the staff. It was desired that they should be free when off duty, and the trust reposed in them was not abused. The orderlies were asked only to take one late pass a week, and they generally fell in with this request; but they appreciated the freedom of the life they might lead, and used to say how lovely it was to be able to go out without being asked where you were going to. Some supervision and some advice were given to those who were younger and less experienced; but the absence of rules and regulations was insisted on, and girls who could not do without them, were advised to return to their mothers. Rumour in the main office had it that the Doctor-in-Charge disapproved of mothers and of marriage, and that you should keep your mother from her, and never, never on any account allow your parents to write to her. The fact was that, acting on the principle that they were adult people, doing responsible work, the Doctor-in-Charge did not write to their parents without their knowledge, and whenever a letter came from parents, even though it contained a request for secrecy, the orderly in question was invited to come and discuss it. From the Doctor-in-Charge's point of view, it was impossible to treat these young women as children, or carry on a correspondence which concerned them without their knowledge, and they would have had little confidence in a chief who acted in such a manner.

It was strange how the kindest of parents thought it proper to control the actions of women well over age, and how younger brothers, uncles, brothers-in-law and the family doctor would think that they had a right to interfere in her business, and would invite the Doctor-in-Charge or the Matron to conspire with them. One could not help sympathising with healthy girls who were made to relinquish the work in which they were successful, and a life which they enjoyed, because ' Mother was dull at home ' or ' Father likes to have his girls with him in the evenings,' or 'She has been away long enough.' No one could blame the girls so coerced if they were bitter and discontented, or the others if they 'strictly forbade' their mothers to interfere. But on the other hand, there were parents whose self-sacrifice and devotion equalled that of their daughters. They gave them their freedom generously, watching them develop with pride, and finding compensation in their happiness and in the knowledge that they were successful and appreciated.

From time to time, an effort was made to interest the orderlies in public questions and to educate their communal sense ; but they viewed these attempts as mild peculiarities on the part of those senior persons who made them, and, smiling and polite, they discouraged them.

In January 1918, the Bill enfranchising women passed the House of Lords, and early the next morning the Doctor-in-Charge was on the steps of her office. She made known to Sergt. Robertson her desire to have the flags run up.

'Certainly doctor,' he replied. And then hesitated.

'I was not aware, Doctor, that it was any special occasion.'

The significance of the occasion was explained

to him, and the whole place was soon gay with bunting.

The young women viewed this celebration with some amusement. They were kind about it, and a little patronising in their congratulations. 'I am so glad your bill has passed all right'; 'It is awfully nice your bill is through'; 'Simply topping about your bill'; said the potential voters, pleased that the older members of the community should have obtained something they desired, and personally quite untouched by their possible share in it.

The beautiful spirit which dominated the staff pervaded the hospital. It was inspiring and uplifting, uniting every one in loyalty and affection, and triumphing over all difficulties and all sorrows. It was the spirit of hope and youth and courage; the spirit which breathed charity for each other and success for all.

When Dr. Louisa Woodcock was dying, she sent her love to Endell Street. 'It is a nice place,' she said, 'a nice spirit.' And then, 'Spirit is the thing that counts.'

It counted, as year succeeded year, and effort had to be multiplied and sacrifice prolonged. It kept the women loyal and generous, harmonious and disciplined. No one came there without being sensible of the spirit of the place, and no one left without being touched by it.

The health of the staff was good on the whole. In 1916, measles claimed a number of victims; but when once disinfection by means of the steam spray was introduced, the rate of sickness was kept very low. During the second influenza epidemic in 1919, only twenty-two persons out of a staff of a hundred and eighty-four were laid low, and this at a time when every one was exposed to infection and was working very hard.

The hospital did not escape without having to mourn the loss of more than one comrade. In January 1918, Miss Eva Prior passed away, dying of Vincent's Angina after a tragic forty-eight hours' illness. She was in the second year of her service, and loved by every one for her sweet disposition and her strength of character. It was the first tragedy. In July 1918, at a time of high pressure and great anxiety, Miss Gladys E. Morrison developed influenza and pneumonia and died, in spite of all that nurses and doctors could do. She was one of those who joined the hospital when it opened, and she had just completed three years continuous and splendid service. Her long association with the hospital had made her part of it, and her many

friends and admirers missed her sadly. Miss
Helen Wilks, who had been one of the assistants
in the Pathological Laboratory, died at home
on January 15th, 1919, of appendicitis, after
many weeks of illness. She was only eighteen
and full of promise. Dr. Elizabeth Wilks, her
mother, wrote :

Endell Street was the great time of her life. She
loved the place and was completely happy. She was
sixteen and a half when Dr. Murray agreed to take her.
We wanted her to continue her studies, thinking her too
young for war work, but she was absolutely determined
to take her part . . . It was completely successful,
and we always felt so thankful that we agreed to her
doing what she wanted to do ; for the last eighteen
months were lived with intense enthusiasm and satisfaction.

In February 1919, Miss Joan Palmes succumbed
to influenza and pneumonia, her death casting
a sad gloom over the hospital. Although, for
family reasons, her service had not been continuous, she had been a member of the staff since
1915. She had a most endearing personality,
gay and courageous and considerate for others.
In the same year Miss Mary Graham died,
away from the hospital, to the great sorrow and
regret of all who knew her.
In a small community, so united and so friendly

as Endell Street, tragedies like these were deeply felt, and those who fell were not forgotten. When Dr. Woodcock died, her funeral took place from Christ Church, Endell Street. And in January 1918, when Dr. Elizabeth Garrett Anderson died, a memorial service for her was held there also. So each fallen comrade was honoured in the church, a guard of honour standing round her, and her comrades forming the choir which gave the Nunc Dimittis. Then, following in sad procession, they stood round her in the square and with sorrowful hearts, took their last farewell. Their feeling was voiced in the paragraph which appeared in ' Orders for the Day ' :

It is with the deepest sorrow and regret that I have to record the death on active service, at this hospital of . . . .

She was our comrade and fellow-worker. She leaves in our hearts a fine memory of one who gave generous and tender service to those who suffered, of one whom we admired and trusted because she responded with courage and devotion to the call of her country.

Our united sympathy will go out to her mother and to those who love and mourn her.

From her work, her example and her sacrifice let us draw fresh inspiration and fresh courage. Let us also put Duty first, as she did. Let us strive to give more, to do more, to sacrifice more, in memory and for the sake of our lost comrade.

In April of 1919, the Doctor-in-Charge was informed that the hospital would be required until the autumn, and arrangements for staffing it for this further period had to be considered.

It was reluctantly decided to demobilise the greater number of the nursing orderlies. The presence of so many young people, however delightful, had always been a heavy responsibility, and the dread of serious illness occurring amongst them again was ever present. Many of them were tired ; others were young and immature ; and since the pressing need for their services no longer existed, it was felt that they should not be subjected to the strain of another six months' work. Only a few of them wished to go, and the motive which prompted those in authority was probably not appreciated, even if it were understood ; but the wisdom of the decision was undoubted. The sorrow and regret at parting was mutual : it was the first step towards disintegration ; and their fellow-workers and the hospital missed them sorely.

The senior nursing orderlies, who remained by their own wish, were supplemented in the wards by R.A.M.C. men, of whom plenty were available then. Their want of training and want of interest in the work made them poor substitutes for the girls who had left.

> Time takes them home that we loved, fair names and
> famous,
> To the soft long sleep, to the broad sweet bosom of death;
> But the flower of their souls he shall take not away to
> shame us,
> Nor the lips lack song for ever that now lack breath.
> For with us shall the music and perfume that die not dwell,
> Though the dead to our dead bid welcome, and we farewell.

CHAPTER VI

THOSE WHO MADE THE WHEELS GO ROUND

IN such a community, one of the most difficult
offices to fill successfully was that of chaplain;
for it is not always possible to combine a voca-
tion for the sick with a sympathetic understanding
of young men and women. The chaplain's work
was solitary and lacked the stimulus of companionship, which was so helpful to the doctors;
and it cannot be denied that a large proportion
of the patients were more interested in the quality
of the surgeons than of the parsons. The efforts
of the Church of England chaplains were supplemented by chaplains of other denominations,
but these only visited the wards and did not
give their whole time to the hospital.

Five chaplains were appointed in succession
to Endell Street, but, except the Rev. Edward
Wells, none of them remained there for any
length of time. Mr. Wells's close and happy
association with the hospital continued for more
than two years and was only terminated in 1919

by his decision to accept a living. From time to time, a locum tenens came for holiday duty or during an interregnum ; but the duties were not easy, and the young and inexperienced men who were sent must often have felt discouraged.

The attitude of the soldier to the chaplain was one of shyness or embarrassment. He was unwilling to be seen talking long with him because other men might tease him about it. Every new chaplain approached him in a different way —some with assumed confidence, some with a brotherly bluffness, some with diffidence. They seemed to find it as hard to be natural as he did. One of them who laid his hand on the patients' heads and stroked their faces, ruined his own cause by the discomfort he caused them. A convalescent, speaking of him, said, ' I am sure he speaks beautifully, but I never could listen : I was so afraid he was going to kiss me.' And the fear was not unfounded ; for in his earnestness, the parson used to bend nearer and nearer, till the men became so nervous that they almost screamed.

Visits out of ordinary hours had a terrifying effect upon the seriously ill, and the wrath of Heaven, in the form of the Chief Surgeon, overtook one chaplain who ventured to disturb a

case she was specially concerned about at eleven
o'clock at night and again at seven in the morning.

Private Stephens, white and trembling, asked :
' Doctor, is it true I am dying ? '

' No, you 're not going to die.   Who said you
were ? '

He rejoined, with tears, ' Chaplain says I must
be prepared ; but I 'd rather trust in you, Doctor.'

Which he did, with the best result.

The visiting of the acutely ill required judg-
ment ; for if it caused fear and excitement
instead of comfort, it could be harmful ; and at
times both Sister and doctor might be anxious
to ward off the chaplain's visit, and yet hesitate
to interfere with his prerogative.

Under Army Orders, church parade was compulsory.   It was unfortunate that it was almost
the only thing which was compulsory at Endell
Street.   In church, the men sat rigidly during
the sermons, their eyes fixed on the preacher
with an appearance of attention, which must
have been very helpful to him.   The methods of
preaching varied with the chaplains.   Those who
were young, favoured local colour.   The Bible
would be referred to as a trenching tool ; the
Prayer Book as an enamelled mug, and the
Twelve Apostles were termed staff officers.   Stories

of the piety of men in the trenches or other hospitals were given and letters from men to the chaplain were often quoted. One preacher was fond of inventing allegories, and conversations between himself and imaginary soldiers, which mystified the men very much. And another who was in favour of Women's Suffrage, preached on the 'New Womanhood,' and exhorted his hearers not to regard those in charge of the hospital as 'playthings,' but as 'their own equals in every respect'; the women being for the time in the position of the men's superior officers !

In the summer of 1919, an Education officer was added to the staff of the hospital, and a few of the men were persuaded to take classes. The first of these officers was unfortunate in having a hesitating, uncertain manner and a bad delivery, which made the men call him 'Mr. Er-er.' The second was very deaf. As a rule, the patients showed little desire to study anything, and only about two per cent. welcomed the scheme, on which the country was spending such enormous sums of money. Teachers in every branch of knowledge were produced. One came to teach shorthand ; another, book-keeping ; others, history, German, singing, or typewriting. The Jewish men were the most anxious for lessons,

STRETCHER-BEARERS AND SERGEANT-MAJOR HARRIS

(Page 218)

(Photo, Reginald Haines)

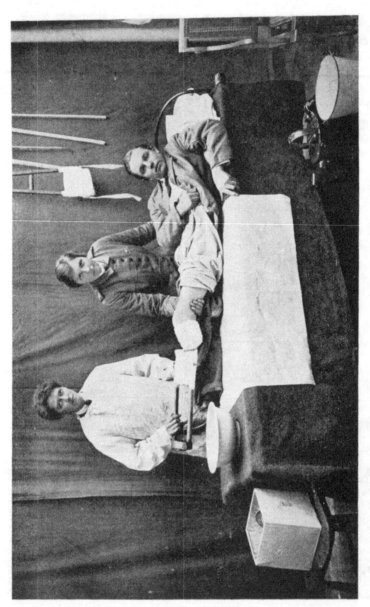

QUARTERMASTER CAMPBELL AND ORDERLY COOK MAKE PLASTER PYLONS

(Photo, Reginald Haines)

but they preferred instruction in voice-production
or singing, and one wished the army to train
him for the operatic stage. The attempt was
not very successful. It did not equal the real
education which the librarian had carried on
during the years that had gone before.

The Hospital was more than fortunate in its
R.A.M.C. detachment, which, though small, was
excellent of its kind. Sergt.-major Harris was in
charge of it from August 1915, until his demobilisation in July 1919. When he was promoted
to the rank of corporal and sent to Endell Street,
his friends in the 35th Company R.A.M.C.
kindly prophesied failure and disaster; but he
remained there for four years as one of the pillars
of the hospital. His experience had been gained
in the St. John's Ambulance Brigade and in the
South African War, and he had not had the
advantage of any training in the work of a warrant
officer. However, his sense of responsibility and
his devotion to duty overcame all obstacles, and
his value to the hospital grew with his rapid
promotion. There were occasions on which
neither the Doctor-in-Charge nor he felt sure
of the correct procedure, and then they would
shut themselves up in her office with ' King's
Regulations ' and ' Regulations for the R.A.M.C.,'

and make a careful study of those wonderful and
intricate volumes. Emerging later, with minds
made up, they pursued the line of action decided
upon, with an air of confidence and custom,
very impressive to all who witnessed it.

In the sergt.-major, the medical staff had a
loyal supporter, who never failed to back up
their authority. He adopted the hospital; took
it to his heart; and often sacrificed Mrs. Harris
and his own leisure to its service. When women
were added to his detachment he trained and
drilled them, and guarded them in a manner
almost paternal. In the sergeants' mess of the
35th Company R.A.M.C., which he visited occasionally, he upheld the credit of his hospital
and of his mixed Company. After such visits,
he would tell the Doctor-in-Charge interesting
details, chiefly about the discipline in other
hospitals, where men habitually stayed out all
night, and where lists of forty or sixty defaulters
were of daily occurrence. 'Nothing like that
here, Doctor,' he would say, with pardonable
self-congratulation.

He was assisted and supported in his duties
by Sergt. Robertson, who began as a private in
1915, and whose reliability and excellence soon
brought him promotion. His good nature was

unfailing. He believed that the Endell Street
Hospital showed the way to all others, and his
chivalry towards women, whether working under
him or as his officers, never failed ; his avuncular
manner included them all.

When the hospital opened, Privates Bishop,
Price, and Hedges, who had been in France with
the Corps, and who had enlisted in February
1915, were transferred to the 35th Company
R.A.M.C., and included in the Endell Street
detachment. The help of such experienced nurses
in the first year was invaluable and their places
were always in the serious wards, where the
heaviest cases and the greatest need of skill
were to be found. Later, when all men of class
' A ' were sent abroad, they found wider fields
of usefulness and more thrilling experiences in
France and in the East.

Corpl. Musselbrook was theatre orderly. Under
the training of the Chief Surgeon and Sister,
he had become very expert in his duties, when
to every one's regret he was suddenly called in
and sent, with several hundred other R.A.M.C.
men, to be trained and transferred into an in-
fantry regiment. He took with him a document
certifying him to be a trained theatre orderly ;
and on the strength of this, he subsequently

got back into the R.A.M.C. and was sent to
Salonika and Russia. On his return to England
in 1919, he came to Endell Street and related
his experiences and successes. He described his
feelings when he went to a hospital in Salonika
and was detailed for duty in the operating theatre.
How the major, in his apron, holding out his
gloved hands, stood silently watching him arrange
the patient; how he himself perspired with
anxiety, as he placed the hands and folded the
clothing; and how suddenly he was asked:
'Where have you been?' When he replied
that he had been at Endell Street, it was a joy
to find that the major had been there too, and
that he shared Corpl. Musselbrook's admiration
for that place and for its women surgeons.
Through all the months that followed, he had
one important post after another, attributing
his success to the early training and to the document, which he always kept on him.

Corpl. Washington succeeded him in the operating theatre, and soon equalled him in skill and
keenness, remaining at his post through several
years of pressure. He was a favourite with the
rest of the staff, and on summer mornings, when
ices were sold in the canteen, Orderly Tanner
might be met slowly ascending the stairs, con-

suming an ice with her right hand and carrying
another for Washington in her left.

The duties of the R.A.M.C. included the care
of the intoxicated men who were constantly
brought in by the police or by the London County
Council ambulances.

These ambulances were staffed by a fine set
of young women, whose serviceable uniform and
alert, well-drilled bearing were a credit to their
service. It was a pleasure, when the ambulance
turned into the square, to see these active girls,
in their navy blue suits of breeches and tunic,
swing themselves off the car, throw the doors
open, unload and bear the stretcher with its
burden to the casualty room. If they thought
that the N.C.O. on duty might be chary of receiving a case of drunkenness—for, strictly speaking, unless otherwise injured, such cases should
not have been brought to the hospital—they
were clever in finding another diagnosis : ' Case
of drugging,' they would cry confidently, tip
the man on to a couch and be off in a whirl of
wheels and blue legs, before the N.C.O. could
stop them. More often they favoured fractures,
and their cases would arrive bound in first-aid
splints or with collar bones duly bandaged. When
splints and bandages were unfastened, it was

not uncommon to have the injured man make violent use of his arms and legs.

The Y.M.C.A. huts also were too kind to diagnose drunkenness, and many a time the hospital sent for cases described by their workers as 'serious' or 'immediate,' only to find them 'fighting drunk.' The huts always seemed to postpone dealing with such cases until late at night, and many an uproar arose in the Johnny Walker Ward when the sergt.-major asked these 'serious' cases to show their 'passes.' Men with 'both collar bones broken' were known to attack him with their fists! Some put their feet through the panels of the door, and others their heads through the window-panes; and the peace of the hospital was so often disturbed that the Doctor-in-Charge finally reported the matter to the Command. Her report included as instances an account of one man who 'bit a policeman and struck the sergt.-major,' and of another, supposed to have a dislocated shoulder, who arrived at 10 P.M. 'As it was a Sunday,' she wrote, 'some of the staff were off duty, and there were only the sergt-.major and a dwarf, and a man with a wasted arm to deal with him.' For in 1917 the physique of the R.A.M.C. was very poor.

There were men who became habitués of the Johnny Walker Ward, for they knew enough to simulate fits when in the hands of the police, and these symptoms would insure that they were taken to the nearest hospital. One of these, who was well known to the doctors, was quieting down after the departure of the police, and the doctor sent for lemonade for him. He took a long pull at the mug, and then looked up at her, and with a regretful sigh said :

'Och ! Dochter, jist think ef it was beer ! '

Many half-intoxicated men had to be admitted to the wards for slight or serious injuries ; for they jumped from windows or fell down areas in their attempts to evade the police ; and the nurses and orderlies became more or less accustomed to looking after them. A voluntary worker at a railway station, thinking that a man in this state was really ill, brought him to the hospital, where he was detained for the night. Not being very busy, the voluntary worker called next morning, full of kind intentions, and was able to conduct the man to the railway station. He wrote afterwards, complaining that the gate officer 'was not by any means sympathetic' about the poor fellow ; which in the circumstances may have been natural, for his case was not exceptional.

When the women orderlies were demobilised in 1919, the male detachment was increased. The men who were sent to the hospital were mostly infantrymen, who for some disability had been transferred to the R.A.M.C. They had had no training, and as a rule they had little liking for ward work, and when put on night duty, they firmly believed that they were entitled to a certain number of hours sleep at night, and to the indignation of the Sisters, were found rolled in rugs on empty beds. It was a rude change, after being accustomed to the ways of the intelligent, gentle young women, to go to a ward at night and ask if a case, newly operated upon, was comfortable, and to be told by a stableman in khaki, 'T' y'ung chaap in t' carner be 'eavin' a bit.' From which it was inferred that the patient was somewhat sick.

The mysteries of hospital life and Sisters' orders were new to them. One of them, being instructed to shave the leg of a patient going up for operation, was greatly puzzled. 'Shave him very close,' said the Sister. 'You must not leave a single hair anywhere.' The orderly's knowledge of asepsis was meagre. He had never heard that legs or arms required shaving; but wishing to carry out his instructions, he attacked the man's face with energy : strictly obedient, he insisted upon removing his moustache ; and so clean did he make his shave that the patient was found sitting up wiping blood from his chin with cotton-wool ; but his leg remained unprepared.

There is always some one behind the scenes who plays an important part in making the wheels go smoothly, some one who works hard and gets no kudos ; and this was so at Endell Street also. There was a band of some twenty-eight or thirty women, referred to on the pay-sheet as ' cleaners ' and by most people as ' char-ladies,' who cleaned and scrubbed and swept and washed-up, day in and day out, year after year. It is impossible to estimate the value of faithful, continuous service of this sort. The cessation of it is demoralising in an institution, for every one's comfort depends upon it. So the char-ladies never failed to come. Labouring patiently, they learnt to love the hospital and to regard it as their own. And on the anniversary of their third year of continuous service, the hospital fêted them. A small presentation was made to each one ; they were appraised by the C.O. in a speech which ' went right through you and was felt in yer very bones,' and cheered by the assembled patients.

P

Working well together, the staff could also
play together; and sometimes a dance would be
given, into which they threw themselves with
delight. Every one came to it—the char-ladies
too; and for once in their lives, these hard-
worked, toil-worn women flung care and husband
and family aside, and gave themselves up to
pleasure. Some yielded to the novelty of wearing men's clothes and appeared in khaki or blue,
as jockeys or as workmen, dancing all night,
enjoying the supper and the speeches, and
looking back on it afterwards as ' a little glimpse
of 'Eaving.'

The R.A.M.C. gleefully decorated the recreation room and polished the floor, and then arrived
disguised as niggers, cowboys, or nurses, led by
the Sergt.-major dressed as a ' lady doctor.'

The Sisters, the masseuses, and the orderlies
were well known to the assistants at Clarkson's
and Simpson's, whose shops they ransacked
periodically. Every kind of dress was worn.
' Little Bits of Fluff ' and cavaliers, pages, sailors,
officers, ballet girls; early Victorian ladies jostled
doctors in Plantagenet costumes, doctors as
Turkish houris, as pierrots or as navvies. Colonel
and Mrs. Dug-out—the one exuberant in kilt
and plaid, with fierce red whiskers; the other

clinging and elegant, in lace cap and mittens—
received the guests and joined in the dance.
The invitation to sit down to supper was greeted
with loud cheers by the guests, so was the Colonel's
speech ; and the toast of ' The Hospital ' was
drunk with Highland honours and much acclamation. There never were such dances as those.
Youth, in its beauty and happiness, was at its
best.

No record of Endell Street would be complete
which did not mention ' Keogh Garrett.' At
the age of six months, he sat on the office table,
asking for approval : a rather weak puppy,
with a beautiful head, neat pointed ears and a
manner which won all hearts. Once assured of
his position, he grew more attractive every day ;
and a chorus of praise and adulation was wont
to follow him as he passed—a dainty little aris-
tocrat, full of character, full of idiosyncrasies,
trotting at the heel of the Chief Surgeon, lying
down before those he loved, turning a deaf ear
and a white eye to those he did not favour.
Affectionate to Sister Lawrence, who massaged
his weak forelegs, adoring the Quartermaster,
he was reticent and dignified towards the patients,
failing to notice their friendly advances, but
remonstrating with any man not in khaki or

blue who entered the square. Outside, in park or street, he would recognise and run to greet the hospital uniform. To this day a floating veil attracts him, and he will do homage to unknown nurses.

The long hours that his family spent in the operating theatre tried him, and as the afternoon waned, he would come upstairs and lie with his nose on his paw just outside the door. He knew he must not enter and cross that shining surface of floor; but he also knew that it mattered less about the floor if the Sister was at tea. What hours he spent on the table in the office window, watching the lift by which friends came back to his world again; how many muddy footprints he left on official documents, and how many colonels he growled at, from his safe retreat on the blotting-paper!

For the sake of companionship, a little ball of white fluff with the blackest of black eyes and nose was added to the staff; and as they grew older, they became wonderfully possessive. William was every one's friend—a veritable cupboard lover and wheedler. He had an unsubdued and boisterous spirit.

How naughty they were to the cats of Soho, who sought a refuge in the hospital precincts,

and how rude to the Matron's dog, whose lineage
they persistently insulted.   On their walks abroad,
they excited admiration and constant reference
to Buchanan's Whisky.   Elderly gentlemen,
tightly buttoned into majors' tunics, would
journey the whole length of a railway car, swing-
ing perilously on the straps, to bend over their
guardian and chuckle, 'Black and white!'   The
patients thought they must be brothers, regardless of the difference of breed; and some even
thought them the sons of Matron's 'Bully';
while the *Daily Mail*, describing a historic scene,
referred to them as 'Black and white Airedales.'
Garrett had all the dignity and airs of Dog-in-
Charge.   William was the little friend of all the
world, and they accepted their position as the
pets and mascots of the hospital.

CHAPTER VII

THE POSITION OF WOMEN UNDER THE WAR OFFICE

In the Spring of 1916, Sir Alfred Keogh called for forty women doctors to replace men in the hospitals of Malta. It was already a well-known fact that the soldier and the woman doctor were compatibles, and the outcry which had greeted the establishment of the Military Hospital, Endell Street, was not repeated. Out of her experience as an army surgeon, Dr. Garrett Anderson wrote to those who were engaged in recruiting these doctors, urging that an effort should be made to secure temporary rank as officers for them, and that they should ask to be formed into a uniformed corps attached to the R.A.M.C. She pointed out that as they were proceeding abroad and were to be distributed among the various hospitals, they would be working with R.A.M.C. officers, and that they would be at a disadvantage professionally if they had not the same status and position as their men colleagues.

Her advice was not taken, and the medical

230

women left England in mufti. They were not
graded, nor paid at officers' rates, but were given
a flat rate which made no allowance for seniority.
These terms, once accepted, were imposed, in
spite of protest, upon all the medical women—
except those at Endell Street—who subsequently
served in hospitals and camps at home or abroad
under the War Office. They did fine work in
Malta, Egypt, Salonika, India, and in France
with the Q.M.A.A.C. At least four hundred of
them gave of their best in the service of the sick
and wounded, carrying on courageously and
generously, although the conditions under which
they had taken service often proved difficult
and humiliating.

The Army's need of women's service grew
greater every day, and the War Office was forced
to consider the necessity of introducing them
widely into hospitals and camps, as dispensers,
storekeepers, cooks, and motor-drivers. In November 1916, a deputation of Red Cross ladies,
headed by Dame Katherine Furse, visited the
Doctor-in-Charge, to inquire into the work done
by women who had replaced men at Endell
Street, and to discuss the formation of a new
section of V.A.D.'s for general service. The
uniform of the Women's Hospital Corps was

highly approved by the deputation as a practical service dress, and when a letter was received asking for the name of the maker, the Doctor-in-Charge thought it advisable to request in writing that it might not be too closely copied. In her reply Dame Katherine Furse wrote :

Would a different colour, style and absence of veil on cap and black shoes and stockings, be sufficient protection ? . . . It would be iniquitous to copy your uniform, which is very much respected by all of us here.

The writer went on to ask questions as to the physical fitness of women for the work it was proposed that they should do.

The Doctor-in-Charge was also asked to give evidence before a Committee of Enquiry which met in December under the auspices of the Board of Education, with a view to determining the capacity of women as substitutes for men. She was actively questioned by the members of the Committee on the subject of stretcher-bearing by women, and offered to arrange a demonstration, so that they might see how well-trained women could acquit themselves in this work.

A few weeks later, Dr. Chalmers Watson, C.B.E., engaged in the organisation of the Q.M.A.A.C., and many long talks over formations and detail were held in the doctor's sitting-room upstairs,

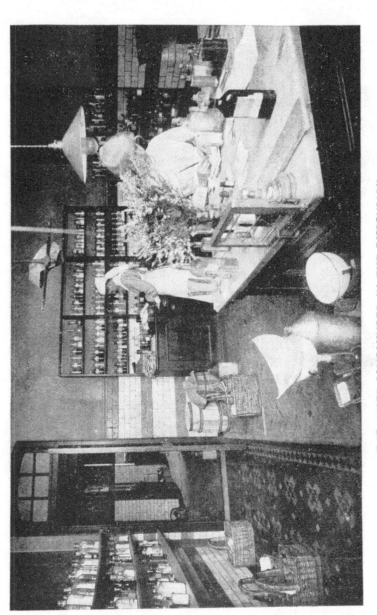

(Photo, Reginald Haines)

THE CHIEF COMPOUNDER IN THE DISPENSARY

(Page 232)

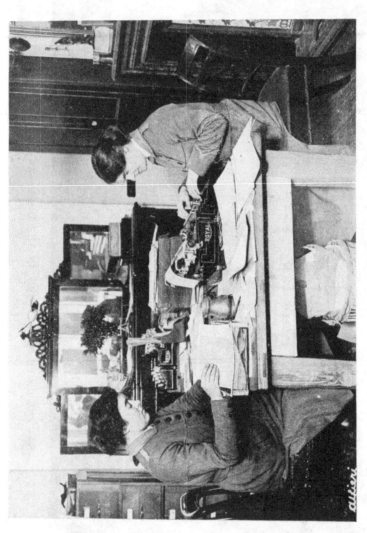

THE CHIEF CLERK IN THE OFFICE

(Page 233)

(*Photo, Alfieri*)

when Dr. Chalmers Watson's ideas on uniforms and her views on discipline and regulations came in for some friendly criticism. It was at Endell Street, too, that she and Dame Helen Gwynne Vaughan were first made known to each other, and it was from the same quarter that she drew some of the early members of her corps. In the desire to help the new service, the Doctor-in-Charge set free Miss Ethel Thomas, the Steward, and Miss Doreen Allen, the Assistant Steward, that they might take administrative posts in the Q.M.A.A.C. Afterwards she always maintained that their success in that corps was due, not so much to their own ability and exceptional qualities, as to the training which they had received at Endell Street.

Dr. Chalmers Watson steered the Q.M.A.A.C. through the shoal of vexatious delays and difficulties which beset its early days with great skill, and she and Dr. Laura Sandeman made a gallant struggle to procure for the women doctors serving with it a position and terms equal to those granted to men.

The first detachments of Q.M.A.A.C. were hurried overseas in the early summer of 1917, and as was only natural, a demand for hospital accommodation arose almost at once. In August,

the Deputy Director of Medical Services, finding
himself at a loss how to meet this demand, approached the Doctor-in-Charge and asked whether
Endell Street could make temporary accommodation for women returning from France. The
arrangement of the building did not lend itself
easily to this purpose, but his request was met
most willingly, and the top floor of one of the
blocks was made ready for their reception. The
situation was complicated by an order from the
War Office to set aside two beds for officials of
the corps.

At first a little room on the Women's floor
was adapted for these ladies; but an order was
shortly received to make room for women requiring to be segregated, and the little room
was no longer available for general use. Small
rooms on other floors were very seldom empty,
and in these circumstances the only beds which
could be offered to officials were those in cur-
tained cubicles in the general ward, which were
used in sickness by the Sisters of the hospital.
The ladies objected to this accommodation even
temporarily, and they were certainly entitled
to better quarters; but they were apt to lay
the blame for a situation over which it had no
control on the hospital, instead of on the Army

Medical Department. After frequent representations from the Doctor-in-Charge, extending
over nine months, instructions were given for
the reception of officials elsewhere ; but in the
meantime irate administrators, arriving in the
middle of the night and refusing to make use
of the only empty bed in the hospital, were sometimes a real difficulty.

The Q.M.A.A.C. Hospital at Isleworth was not
opened till the end of January 1919, and the
'temporary accommodation' at Endell Street was
required for more than two years. The other
women's services found it convenient to use it,
and members of the G.S.V.A.D., the W.R.N.S.,
N.A.C.B., W.R.A.F., and W.L., found a resting
place there. Ladies were admitted from overseas and the East, with babies, nurses, governesses,
and occasionally husbands ; while, under the
heading of ' civilians,' women who were working
in France with the Y.M.C.A., the Soldiers'
Christian Union, the Expeditionary Force Canteens, the Lena Ashwell Concert Parties, and
officers' wives and servants, were also given
hospitality.

While this development in the women's services
was proceeding, the Government was making
increasing demands upon medical women, and

was introducing them in greater numbers into the hospitals at home and abroad. In August 1917, a cable from Lady Chelmsford reached Dr. Garrett Anderson, asking to be informed as to the terms of appointment of doctors at Endell Street, and this was followed by a letter from the Secretary of the Central Committee of the Countess of Dufferin's Fund at Simla. She stated that it had been decided ' that one of the large military hospitals in Bombay should be handed over to women doctors,' and she asked for information and suggestions which might be helpful in organising it. The reply sent gave details of the Endell Street establishment, and urged that the women should undertake the ' entire control and management' of the hospital. It advised, on grounds of economy, that women should be employed as quartermasters and storekeepers, spoke of the ease with which discipline could be maintained by women, and of the help which a good warrant officer could give.

The Indian hospital was established on one of the finest sites in Bombay ; but the charge of the hospital was vested in men, a Colonel and a Registrar being appointed, although women doctors could have filled these posts. The professional work, however, was in the hands of

women, and they made an undoubted success
of it. In 1919 when men were brought home
from India in large numbers, some who had
been in the Women's Hospital at Bombay came
to Endell Street. They said it was 'the only
good hospital they had been to in India,' and
spoke of it and of its doctors with great appreciation and pleasure.

A request for information and help came from
medical women in America during 1918, enclosing
a copy of a resolution which the Women Physicians of California were sending to their Government. The resolution urged

upon the Secretary of War that the services of women
physicians be utilised to the fullest extent by the United
States War Department in the present war ; that opportunities for medical service be given to medical women
equal to the opportunities given to medical men, both
as members of the staffs of base hospitals and otherwise ; and that the women so serving be given the
same rank, title and pay given to men holding equi-
valent positions.

As a result of this petition, the American War
Department communicated with the British War
Office, asking a number of questions concerning
the employment of women doctors. The right
hand of the War Office never seemed to know

what the left hand was doing, and three separate staff officers, each armed with notebook and pencil, called on three separate occasions to obtain the information which the American Government required from the Doctor-in-Charge.

Doctors working for the Army in isolated posts wrote to Endell Street to tell of difficulties or grievances arising out of their anomalous position. They were doing the work of officers and were supposed to exercise the authority of officers, yet they were not officers. In some cases, they were refused first-class travelling warrants and were furnished with third-class 'as for soldiers' families,' while their R.A.M.C. colleagues and the nurses were issued with the former. Or, on the ground that they were 'civilian women,' the right to drive in an army motor-car would be withheld from them ; or they would be excluded from the officers' mess.

One wrote from East Africa, stating that her position had been excellent under a C.O. who allowed her to wear a captain's badge of rank, but that his successor had ordered her to remove it, and she was therefore a discredited person in the hospital to which she was posted. Women working under R.A.M.C. colonels in R.A.M.C.

hospitals were at the mercy of the wisdom or
the prejudices of the officers-in-charge, and the
pin-pricks and little indignities to which they
were often subjected were very unfair. They
were volunteers, in the best sense of the word,
and if their services were accepted at all, no
difference should have been made between them
and the men they worked among.

In a women's unit, internal difficulties like
these did not arise ; but the officer-in-charge
of a military hospital is required to deal with
small offences ; and when the Doctor-in-Charge
' admonished ' defaulters, she was conscious that
her authority would have been greatly strength-
ened if she had been wearing the badges of a
lieut.-colonel. In the casualty room, where men
might not recognise a woman as an officer, the
doctors were sometimes placed at a disadvantage ;
but the good feeling of the N.C.O.'s and the support
which they gave to their medical staff avoided
any real trouble.

Urged thereto by the President of the Medical
Women's Federation, Dr. Garrett Anderson and
Dr. Flora Murray took up the question with the
War Office, and asked for honorary rank or com-
missioned rank for women doctors serving with
H.M. Forces. The Department refused, but it

was interesting to find that many individual officers could see no objection to rank being held by women.

During the weeks of tension and anxiety which preceded the armistice, no further action seemed possible ; but shortly after that event, the medical staff was unanimously in favour of reopening the matter. The campaign started with a letter from Dr. Garrett Anderson to *The Times*. But the Editor suppressed the correspondence which followed, and the doctors therefore circularised the House of Commons. A leaflet entitled ' Bricks without Straw ' was sent out to all Members of Parliament in November 1918. It stated the disabilities complained of by medical women serving under the War Office, and called attention to the action of the Income Tax Commissioners, who had refused their claim to be assessed at the service rate.

Women had been recently enfranchised and the General Election was approaching. The circular received a large and sympathetic response. One member wrote :

As they are doing the same work as men in the military hospitals, I can see no reason why they should not be entitled to the same style or commission . . .

Other members wrote :

There is ample precedent for the grant of honorary
rank to ladies in the Armies of Europe—and seeing that
the practical value of it can be proved in this case, I
think it should be given.

The decision of the Income Tax Commissioners referred
to in your letter to *The Times* must be reversed if the
rank is granted, and should be challenged if the rank is
not granted.

And :

. . . You may rely upon me now and upon all future
occasions to support the demand you make.

And :

There seems to me to be great force in your con-
tention that where a woman doctor has to perform
the duties of a colonel, in authority over a large
number of different sorts of troops in a general military hospital, she should have the advantage which
military rank would give in maintaining discipline among
them.

Altogether sixty-two Members of Parliament
gave definite promises of support and many
others expressed a desire to help. Questions
were asked in the House ; and the amount of
sympathy and interest evinced by Members
were astonishing to those who made the usual
official replies. It was, however, too late in the
session to do more. Parliament was on the point

of dissolving, and every one's thoughts were concerned with the coming election.

When the new House of Commons met in February 1919, the Prime Minister and Mr. Bonar Law were pledged 'to remove all existing inequalities of the law as between men and women.' The doctors circularised the new House without delay, desiring to obtain consideration for their requests before the new Army Act and Finance Act were drafted. The documents forwarded to Members were entitled : ' Memorandum on the position of Women Doctors serving under the War Office,' and ' Application for Relief under Service Rate of Income Tax by Women Doctors serving the War Office.' The first requested that legislation might ' be introduced under the New Army Act to enable women doctors serving under or attached to the War Office to hold Commissions.' The second asked for an alteration in the wording of the Income Tax Act.

In 1915-16, the doctors had claimed to be assessed under the Service Rate of Income Tax, quoting Schedule E, page 2 :

Persons who have served during the year as members of any of the naval or military forces of the Crown, or in service of a naval or military character in connection

with the present war for which payment is made out of
money provided by Parliament . . . special rates of
tax and scales of allowances are applicable to the pay in
connection with any such service.

The Surveyor of Taxes, however, disallowed the
claim, though he could give no reason for doing
so. The matter was referred to the Secretary
of the Board of Inland Revenue in 1916-17,
and without giving any reason, he also informed
them that they were not eligible for the special
rate of tax. In 1917-18, an appeal was heard
by the Income Tax Commissioners, who decided
that ' on the wording of the Section relief could
not be granted,' and advised them to spend a
large sum of money in making an application
to the High Court. All these persons were pro-
fuse in expressions of sympathy, which were
naturally irritating to women who were only
asking for justice. The application to Parliament made a point of asking that relief might
be made retrospective over the years 1914-1919.
This appeal to the House of Commons met with
far less response than the first one had done.
Members who had written almost gushingly
before the general election, forgot to reply at
all ; others thought that everything had been
done which could be done, or pointed out that

the War was over; and when unsatisfactory replies to questions were received and friends moved the adjournment of the House, sufficient support was not forthcoming.

The women were supported by the British Medical Association. The matter had been brought before the Naval and Military Sub-Committee, and its members had been unanimously in favour of commissioning medical women.

Although the first point was not conceded, the second was, and the new Income Tax gave women doctors relief under the Service Rate, and allowed them to claim to be refunded, as from the year 1915-16. The staff at Endell Street had learnt to look upon Surveyors and Commissioners as 'oppressors of the poor,' and it was with genuine satisfaction that they forwarded to these sympathetic gentlemen claims for abatement and refund.

In the autumn of 1919, an official circular letter invited the commanding officers of all units and formations to suggest 'amendments' to the Army Act. This gave the Doctor-in-Charge a last opportunity of pleading for equality for women and men, whether as medical officers, nursing orderlies, general service orderlies, clerks,

or storekeepers. And it enabled her to propose
the formation of a reserve of women organised
on territorial lines and available in future emergencies.

Whether her draft ever reached the War Office,
or whether it was buried in some waste-paper
basket on the way, is not known.

CHAPTER VIII

CLOSURE OF THE MILITARY HOSPITAL
ENDELL STREET

GOVERNMENT Departments tend to economise by keeping a careful watch over the salaries of their subordinate staff, and a great deal of correspondence and effort were directed to improve the conditions of pay for various groups of the women employed.

A strenuous attempt was made to obtain better terms for clerks, for the pay given to them in 1915 was not a living wage. Twenty-five shillings a week was considered enough for shorthand typists; and a colonel who was interviewed on the subject refused assistance on the ground that ' the girls in his office got no more, and they looked alright.' After weeks of letter writing, the pay was raised to twenty-six shillings, with overtime at ninepence an hour ; and gradually it was pushed up for all grades of Government clerks. When a bonus for clerks was introduced, the men received four shillings a week and the

women two shillings, although they were doing
the same work. The weekly salary finally reached
thirty-nine shillings and forty-five shillings, but
the rate was always below that paid by civilian
employers, and the Government was in the position of exploiting the patriotism and generous
feeling of the women who worked for it.

The Quartermaster was graded and paid as a
sergeant-major and the storekeepers as sergeants.
When these officials had given two years' service,
it was requested that the Quartermaster might
be promoted to a higher grade, and as this was
refused because she was a ' civilian,' a claim was
made for authority to draw the bonus for her
and the sergeants to which civilian employees
were entitled. After many weeks of waiting,
the Doctor-in-Charge was informed that these
members of the staff were not civilians. Since
they were paid under Royal Warrant, they were
N.C.O.'s, R.A.M.C., and were entitled to draw
an additional penny a day for each year of
service. Thus, instead of a bonus amounting
to some shillings weekly, the Quartermaster was
allowed to draw an additional 1s. 2d. per week ;
and a similar economy was made in respect of
other members of her staff. Many months later,
when the army bonus and new rates of pay

were introduced, the authorities would fain have designated these officials as 'civilians.' But the letter calling them N.C.O's., R.A.M.C., was very definite, and both they and the medical officers benefited by the new rates.

The files were full of letters about inadequate pay or insufficient allowances, or requests that the staff of Endell Street might come under new rates announced in Army Council Instructions which did not specially mention that hospital. In most cases the requests were granted after long delay, and the arrears which accumulated during the period of negotiation were drawn in a lump sum, and made a pleasant impression of wealth.

A notable instance of procrastination occurred over the cooks' pay, correspondence concerning which spread over eleven months! The cooks all had three or four years of continuous service to their credit; during that period thay had not received any increment, and the bonus granted to 'civilian subordinates' had been refused to them. Then the rate of pay for women engaged in cleaning and in the kitchen work was raised; and the vegetable women and kitchen maids began to draw higher pay than the cooks under whom they worked. It speaks volumes for the

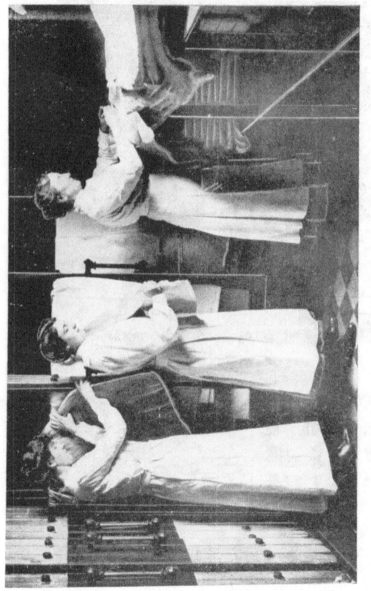

AIRING LINEN

(Photo, Reginald Haines)

(Page 246)

HOSING THE SQUARE

(Photo, Reginald Haines)

(Page 247)

good-feeling and loyalty of the cooks that no unpleasantness occurred over this situation ; and that although readjustment was delayed month after month, everything continued to go smoothly and well. A few weeks before the hospital closed the new rate of pay was settled, and a substantial sum in arrears was available for each one.

It may have been that the new Women's Corps and Services offered a more attractive life to women, or that hospital work began to pall upon them after several years of war ; but it became more difficult to find recruits, and in 1918 a glad welcome was extended to a number of American women who came over to London to serve as orderlies at the Military Hospital, Endell Street. This little group of women was known as the ' Hazard unit ' ; for the work of organising it and sending it to England was due to the energy, resource and friendship of Mrs. Hazard of Syracuse. The American women, though untrained in hospital work and unaccustomed to English life, took up the task before them with great enthusiasm, and proved very useful members of the staff. The hospital was much indebted to Miss Nancy Cook and Miss Marion Dickerman, who gave a year of most valuable service, and whose happy personalities endeared them to all those with whom they came in contact.

The problem of resting the orderly staff was always important, and as the years passed, it became more pressing. The holidays allowed under the terms of appointment were very insufficient, and it was essential to give each one a full month's leave in the summer, if they were to keep well and fit for the work. This could only be done if other girls could be found to take their places temporarily; for the summer was always the busiest time of the year. An appeal for temporary workers was sent to a number of the women's colleges and girls' schools, and in 1917 and 1918 a very cordial response was met with.

During the vacation, students from the London School of Medicine for Women came in large numbers to work in the wards and laboratories and operating theatre. Teachers from the women's colleges at Oxford and Cambridge and from girls' schools gave up a month or a fortnight of their hard-earned rest to relieve the hospital orderlies. Older girls came by tens from Roedean School for girls to take up administrative or clerical work or to be general duties orderlies. Wycombe Abbey sent its contingent, and friends and younger sisters volunteered to help also. The scheme was a great success : the regular orderlies appreciated the good holiday and came back better for it, and the substitutes enjoyed the novelty of the work and surroundings, and learnt much that was useful to themselves. Sunburnt, muscular schoolgirls appeared to find great pleasure in conveying stores and linen about the hospital, and their good spirits were a delightful asset. They took an interest too, in the personnel and customs of the hospital, and were wont to carry on conversations about them in loud tones, which were very amusing to those who could not help overhearing them.

A dormitory which three Roedean girls and an Endell Street orderly were using was very close to the rooms occupied by Dr. Flora Murray and Dr. Garrett Anderson. One summer night, as the babel of voices in the residential quarters died down, the piercing conversation close at hand attracted their attention.

1st Roedean : ' Do you like Dr. Murray ? '

2nd Roedean : ' No, I don't think I do.'

1st Roedean : ' Why don't you like her ? '

2nd Roedean : ' Oh, I don't know. I don't think I like her manner.'

3rd Roedean : ' Have you ever spoken to her ? '

2nd Roedean : ' Yes, I have, once.'

1st Roedean : ' What does she do ? '

Orderly : ' Oh, she sits in that office.'

1st Roedean : ' Do you like Dr. Anderson ? '

2nd Roedean : ' Yes, I like her awfully.'

3rd Roedean : ' Have you ever spoken to her ? '

2nd Roedean : ' Oh no, I 've never spoken to her.'

1st Roedean : ' What does she do ? '

Orderly : ' Oh, she does all the operations.'

Roedean in chorus : ' Oh ! how horrible ! '

Warning voice from room above : ' Campbell ! '

Orderly : ' Yes.'

Voice : ' *They* can hear every word you say.'

The silence which fell was almost as penetrating as the voices had been.

But while they retained their independence of mind and their vivacity, they gave very real service to the hospital ; and the Doctor-in-Charge and the Matron were not less grateful than the orderlies who owed so much to the students and others who set them temporarily free.

During the winter months which followed the Armistice there was little change in the work coming into the hospital. Men arrived in large numbers from France and from the East, and the hospital was full to overflowing for Christmas

1918. It was to be the last Christmas at Endell
Street, and the Entertainment Committee and
the staff decided that it was to be the best, and
festivities and gaieties were organised on a special
scale. As the new year advanced, men began
to arrive from every part of the world; the
hospital ships brought them from India, Egypt,
Mesopotamia, Palestine, and Turkey, Salonika
and Russia, Italy and Africa. Some were recovering from wounds; some were repatriated
prisoners of war; and others were suffering from
diseases contracted in the East.

The surgical work became less pressing, and
more wards were set aside for medical patients.
Cases of pneumonia and acute appendicitis were
as frequent as ever, but there was less night
work; the convoys were fewer and came at
reasonably early hours, and there were no air-
raids to get every one out of bed. Innumerable
men on demobilisation leave reported or were
brought in for accidents or illness, and the
'Johnny Walker' Ward was in constant use at
night.

The returning soldier was strangely unmoved
by the countries he had visited, and seemed to
have learnt little of their geography and inhabit-
ants, and to care not at all what became of them.

254 WOMEN'S HOSPITAL CORPS, LONDON

Palestine, perhaps, had interested him most, for
the familiar Biblical stories and names of places
had made it real for him. A Scotsman, who was
wounded two miles distant from Jerusalem,
never ceased to regret that he had not entered
that city. He had been thrilled by the waters
of Jordan and moved by the sight of Gaza and
Beersheba, and it was a bitter disappointment
to be carried back and to miss the Holy City.
Others spoke of the Mount of Olivet and the road
from Jerusalem to Jericho, of Joppa and of
Lebanon, with an interest and an appreciation
which was very different from that shown for
Italy or Greece. But the general feeling was
one of relief at being back in England, combined
with an intense eagerness to be demobilised.

Regulations for demobilisation were issued at
first in pamphlet form, and later as thick books
in more than one volume. They were supplemented by conferences held at Headquarters,
at which most confusing discussions took place,
and the blind attempted to lead the blind to their
mutual embarrassment. The regulations were
amended, altered, or amplified almost week by
week, and the frequent small changes in procedure had to be observed and noted. It was
easy to make a slip among the complicated rules

for the disposal of patients. The men did not themselves understand the regulations for demobilisation, and each one was inclined to think himself entitled to ' get out first,' or failed to see how his position differed from that of his more fortunate neighbour. Convoys of convalescent hospital cases arrived from Russia or Italy or India, all eager to get home, and anxious not to be detained long in the home hospital. The staff applied itself with energy to the task of holding Boards and making up documents, and many were the compliments received from N.C.O.'s and men upon the rapidity with which their demobilisation was completed. Men from various units who were about to be demobilised, or men who had been demobilised, attended by hundreds in the casualty room, for medical examination and report, and the task of examining them and assessing their disabilities made heavy demands on the time of the doctors.

As the summer months passed, the tone of the men in the wards gradually changed. They only wanted to get out of the army : to be rid of discipline, to get back their former work, or to be pensioned. They craved for liberty and plenty of amusement, and above everything they desired to see restrictions of every kind removed.

The inevitable reaction had set in, and they were filled with half-understood desires and a dissatisfaction which they could not explain.

As other hospitals in London closed, their patients were transferred to those that remained open, and many such transfers were sent to Endell Street. Apart from further treatment, which might or might not be required, numbers of these men were ready to be demobilised, others to be invalided ; and many asked to be transferred to the neighbourhood of their own homes. The Scots would wish to be sent to Scotland, the Irish to Ireland, the Welsh to Wales ; and for all such local accommodation was obtained. The tone and manner of men transferred from other hospitals, where discipline was slack, were unpopular with the staff ; but after a few days, the civilising influences of the nurses triumphed and the men adopted more gentle ways. There were times when eighty or a hundred men arrived with the intention of giving trouble, and those in charge found it necessary to exert their authority and take a firm stand. It was especially during these latter months that the work of the doctors would have been much easier if they had been wearing badges of rank.

In October 1919, an order was issued to evacuate

and close the hospital; and though this instruction had been more or less expected, it was nevertheless received with regret; for it meant the termination of the work and the dispersal of those who had been united so long and so happily in the Women's Hospital Corps.

No more convoys came in, and as the disposal of the present cases was systematically proceeded with, the wards gradually fell vacant. There was stock-taking to do and equipment to be returned to store before the nursing staff could be released. Deficiencies and breakages were disclosed, and the unaccountable disappearance of scissors and bath-towels clouded the last days. By the end of the month, the remaining patients had been passed over to other hospitals. The doctors dined together and spent a festive evening at the Alhambra. They held their last staff meeting and separated, with a pleasant sense of work accomplished, many happy memories and the knowledge that the ties of friendship would not be readily broken.

The Matron and Sisters were demobilised, and sadly turned to other work or holidays. The last of the nursing orderlies said farewell, and there remained only the clerks and quarter-

master's staff, with the Doctor-in-Charge, for
the purpose of winding up.

In recognition of their services, six awards of
the Order of the British Empire were made to
doctors, and eleven Royal Red Crosses were bestowed upon the Matron and nursing Sisters.
Members of the Corps who had served in France
were also entitled to receive the 1914 Star, the
British War Medal and the Victory Medal.

Before finally separating, the members of the
Women's Hospital Corps determined to perpetuate
the name of the hospital which had grown so dear
to them all, and it was decided to raise a Com-
memoration Fund and to endow a bed in the
Women's Hospital for Children in Harrow Road.
This hospital was chosen because Dr. Garrett
Anderson, Dr. Flora Murray and Dr. Buckley
were on its staff, and because it aimed at giving
opportunities to women doctors in the study and
practice of children's medicine. Under the able
direction of Dr. Buckley and Dr. Sheppard, an
appeal was issued to all who had worked at Endell
Street and to all who had been patients there;
and within a few months the first £1000 was
subscribed. The response from old patients was
very friendly, and many of them took a great

deal of trouble to collect among their friends and fellow-workmen, and sent substantial contributions.

Private S—— sent 50s. with a letter : ' I have done my best for you. I took the letter you sent me into work with me and some of them agreed to help me, so I made out a paper as you will see and took it round the Firm so you must excuse it being so dirty and would you kindly let me have a letter back to take into work and show my Fellow workmen.'

Private C—— wrote that he had got up a dance. ' I thought I would like to do something towards it, being so good to me while I was in Hospital there, so I have been able to get up a Dance in our village and I am glad to say I had a good company there to help towards it, being for a good cause, so I hope you will accept this order for £5, 9s. 0d.'

Private Cl—— enclosed 14s., with the words : ' I try my best to help you the way I was cared for when I was there.'

A touching letter from the niece of a man who had been killed since his stay in the hospital, said : ' . . . . which my Mother's brother was an inmate for a time wounded, I wish to state that he was killed at Bullecourt in France some few months afterwards. He was my Mother's only brother, and she is now the only one left of the family. She wishes to most heartily thank all who cared and tendered for him whilst he lay so far from home. She also wishes to send a small donation of 2s. 6d. to help a little your grand and God given work.'

The wife of another man who had died sent £1, ' on behalf of my Late Husband . . . who died Feb. 28th, 1919, from Influenza and Lobar Pneumonia after a week's illness. He was just demobed three weeks to the day we buried him. It will be a surprise to those who nursed him at Endell St. He often spoke about it of what they had done for him & the kindness shown to them the sister he said was a mother to him there was no hospital as good as Endell St. to him he had some real good times there & he never forgot them.'

Others became annual subscribers or filled collecting boxes, and their letters showed affectionate remembrance of the staff. ' I was very Thankful for what I had done for me in Endell Street Hospital. And thanks for sending me the Photo of the Staff. As the Doctor is on it what attended me. So I can show it to my Friends.'

And again : ' I was cared for kindly at that

hospital and I was sorry to leave it. I was wounded twice after being at that Hospital but I wasn't cared for anywhere else so kindly as I was at Endell St.'

Contributions came, too, from Australia and New Zealand, from Canada, America, and South Africa ; and during the year 1920, enough money was subscribed to name a second cot after the Military Hospital, Endell Street.

Endell Street was a changed place. The dreary, empty wards, where equipment was collected and counted and checked, were miserable in their loneliness. The busy kitchen was handed over to the R.A.M.C. cook. The girls who remained counted linen and glass and china, or sorted cutlery, furniture, pianos, wheel-chairs, and all the hospital impedimenta. They concentrated on ledgers and registers. They entered and checked and corrected, from morning till night. Romance had gone out of the life and ' Finis ' was written on the walls ; but the old unquenchable cheerfulness still dominated the stores and offices.

The Office of Works invaded the buildings early in November. After that, workmen, who seemed to be always waiting for something or some one, hung round the empty wards and staircases. A discourteous foreman lounged about, with his hands in his pockets, and smoked and spat and pushed his way into the offices without asking permission. The noise in the square became intolerable : carts and vans and motor-lorries came and went constantly ; workmen played football at all hours, and the bell clanged to summon them to and from work. In a confidential moment, an officer at Headquarters said that ' the Office of Works was almost more than flesh and blood could bear.' And the Doctor-in-Charge fully endorsed this opinion.

By the end of November the ledgers and returns were practically finished, and it was possible to demobilise the remaining members of the staff. When they separated, as they did reluctantly and with sorrow, the closure of the hospital was complete.

There was other work for professional people, like doctors and nurses and clerks, to take up ; but the future was blank to the young girls who had been there so long and who were now to be unemployed. They missed the hospital and the hospital life sadly. In many cases there was no special place in the home circles for daughters who had been living away for some years ; those who had experienced the joy of work and of responsibility, had to exchange these for the comparative inactivity of home-life. Parental restrictions had become unfamiliar and now seemed irksome to them; and they found unrelieved amusement a poor substitute for work. Thus they suffered considerably, until they were able to adapt themselves to new conditions or to find new openings.

The Doctor-in-Charge and Miss Draper, the chief compounder, were detained for some weeks longer to supervise the removal of the stores and equipment. Once this was accomplished, their work was finished, and on the 8th January 1920 the buildings were formally handed over.

The Office of Works took final possession of the premises, and devoted them to a different purpose under a quite different name, and 'The Military Hospital, Endell Street,' became a wonderful and cherished memory.

Printed in Great Britain by T. and A. CONSTABLE, Printers to His Majesty, at the Edinburgh University Press.